RAVE REVIEWS FOR **ODD ONE OUT**

"I read *Odd One Out* in two days but got years' worth of good, solid advice, strategies and insights. This is a book that cuts to the chase. Jennifer doesn't spend page after page walking you through various theories, wordy thoughts and ideas; she grabs you and TELLS you what will work by giving you specific tools to help you become a maverick—someone who embraces their ADHD and moves forward in spite of it.

This is a book that will help anyone who has been diagnosed with ADHD, whether it was a month ago or 10 years ago. If you are feeling stuck and unsure as to how to get your life on track, pick up this book, follow her tips, and you too will take charge of your life and begin living it as a warrior. I will be recommending this one to all of my clients!"

• Terry Matlen, ACSW, Author of *Survival Tips for Women with ADHD*
Birmingham, MI, www.ADDconsults.com

"I have purchased just about every single book on ADD management that has been published. After spending hundreds of dollars, I finally found a book that actually makes sense—doesn't make me feel like a 'special needs adult'—and provides a strategy for managing, and more importantly, getting the most out of my ADD!"

• Angela Palmier, Smithton, IL

"In *Odd One Out*, Jen Koretsky has cut through the fluff that ADDers don't have the time or patience for and gets to the real essence of what's needed to get the real benefits from your ADD traits. In her casual, straight talking style of writing she gets to the real essence of what it takes to be more successful, happier and more confident—all because of your ADD, not in spite of it.

Having read just a couple of chapters of this book (in whichever order you fancy!), you will have some of the tools to tap into your brilliance and bring out the true maverick inside you—all in a way that feels comfortable and true to who you are. Highly recommended."

• Sital Ruparelia, London, England, www.AuthenticResourcing.com

"As a newly diagnosed adult with ADD, *Odd One Out* is the absolute BEST book I have read on this subject. Very reader friendly (I read mine cover to cover). It is obvious that Jennifer knows what she is talking about and has been there and done that. This is not just a bunch of helpful tips and tricks; it is real information that you can identify with and put into action. Thanks so much!"

• Rhonda Crowder, St. Charles, IL

"*Odd One Out* was a refreshing and uplifting book. I think I've read every single book about ADD, and this one has definitely been my favorite. It taught me how to think differently about myself and showed me how to work with my ADD instead of against it...which I've been doing for so long! *Odd One Out* has opened up a dialogue with my husband that has truly transformed our marriage, and now I feel like someone else understands me!! Thanks Jennifer for giving me so much hope and encouragement!!"

• Allison Campos, Hubbard, OR

"As a recently diagnosed 53-year-old, I needed a resource that was very practical, useful, and had 'use it today' strategies. This book has these strategies in abundance. As a result, my concept of ADD has changed. I feel much better about myself. And for the first time in many, many years I can see blue skies ahead. I recommend *Odd One Out* to anyone with ADD, it's the best book I've read by far! Thanks Jennifer."

• Brady Oglesbee, Clackamas, OR

"*Odd One Out* is the first book about ADD that made me truly see and feel my ADD as an asset instead of a liability."

• Helga Van Vondelen, Leiden, The Netherlands

"Jennifer Koretsky offers solutions in *Odd One Out* for living with the challenges of ADD. Embracing simplicity, breaking the cycle of over-whelm and better organization through planning the time to plan are straightforward concepts the reader can put into action immediately for results. For ADD outsiders, maverick Koretsky offers a glimpse into life within the world of ADD for better understanding and communi-cation. Not exclusive advice for only those with ADD, her principles for simplification for a happier life are good reading for all."

• Doug Emerson, Lockport, NY, www.profitablehorseman.com

"I had 4 books to read on ADD, and Jennifer's was the only one that I couldn't put down. That was partly due to the friendly writing style and its practical suggestions, eloquently expressed. It was also nice to see that it was done by someone who dealt personally with ADD, and not someone who just treated others for the condition."

• Bill Kemper, Bogart, GA

"*Odd One Out* tells it like it is! Before I read the book, I had taken pride in being called a 'miscreant' by one of my long time co-workers. When I get back to the office I'm going to give back the 'miscreant' description and replace it with 'maverick'!"

• Karen Bick, Dalllas, TX

"I couldn't put the book down! It's so readable, with elegantly pared down prose...there is plenty of information to absorb and your solutions were simple, sensible, and oh so do-able. Thank you so much for this little gem of a book. It is without doubt a clear new voice and an important one in the wobbly world of ADD. I also feel every non-ADDer trying to get a glimpse of what having ADD means should definitely read and contemplate this book."

• Lynn Root, Fort Collins, CO

"*Odd One Out* is a fresh and affirming take on ADD. I found the book encouraging and empowering. The author's personal stories rang very true for me, and her tone and style made me feel like she was talking to me."

• Keith Schleicher, Glen Allen, VA

"*Odd One Out* is fantastic! It's a clear, accurate and extremely helpful book. Each page addressed the problems that I have, and live with daily. I have read a LOT of ADD books over the years. *Odd One Out* is readable, informative, and also is full of practical advice. It is a book that will be helpful in letting me Live out Loud. Thank you so much!"

• Sam Hooker, Federal Way, WA

"Most people think of ADHD as a lack of focus and don't understand the toll it takes to try to keep up with demands of everyday life...This is the first book I have read that really describes the frustration and emotional struggle that can accompany ADHD."

• Linda Cleary, Springfield, MA

"In Jennifer's no holds barred book, she generously shares her own personal and professional stories (the good, the bad and the highly ADD moments) and she shares her own personal strategies for getting through life with ADD.

But it's just not another ADD book! Jennifer tells you why it's ok to have ADD, why being the '*Odd One Out*' can work for you, not against you. She also shares resources and gives you some action plans too! After reading the chapter "Take Control of Your Space and Time", I cleaned my bedroom (a task that had been in my mental list of things to do for months!). If a book can make ME clean, organize and most of all take action then it's worth a read!!!"

• Sandra De Freitas, Author of *Does This Blogsite Make My Wallet Look Fat?* Toronto, ON, Canada, www.TechCoachforCoaches.com

"I bought your book and couldn't put it down. Being a mother with ADD, it hit home, made me laugh, and gave me some good pointers. I passed it to my 28-year-old ADD daughter. I am sure I will be buying another copy to keep for myself."

• Darlene Bradshaw, Ocala, FL

"*Odd One Out* gives hope to those of us who think we are 'different' and gives us a reason to celebrate the way we are. After reading this book, I felt wiser and stronger."

• Gay Anne Ewing, East Hartford, CT

"I have always been an ADDer who gets trapped in an overwhelm cycle which has lead to me not succeeding most of my life although I know that I am highly intelligent. After reading *Odd One Out*, I realized I can break the cycle of overwhelm and do great things in my life.

I am now taking action. I am able for the first time in my entire life to really take control. I realize what I am doing wrong, and most importantly I realize that I am not wrong, it is just that I got into the habit of doing things in the wrong way because I really did not understand me. I would really like to thank you."

• Thulane Akinjide-Obonyo, London, England

"This is the first book a newly diagnosed person should read because you see that there's hope and there's humor in ADD, and knowing that can help you move forward. *Odd One Out* is quick-witted and easy to read. It felt more like having a conversation than reading a book and at times I was laughing out loud. I could relate to so many of her experiences. Jen tells it like it is, and I loved her openness and honesty.

Even though she's an expert, Jen doesn't beat you over the head with information. Her approach is more like 'I've lived it, this is what happens, and these are the strategies and techniques I've developed.' She gives you a clear, easy to follow breakdown of her skills for managing ADD. This book is an outline on how to live every day, and how to live with your Attention Deficit Disorder. This book is fabulous across the board!"

• Cindy Giardina, ADHD Coach and ADHD Book Club Leader Wayne, NJ,
www.kaleidoscope-coaching.com, www.adhdbookclub.com

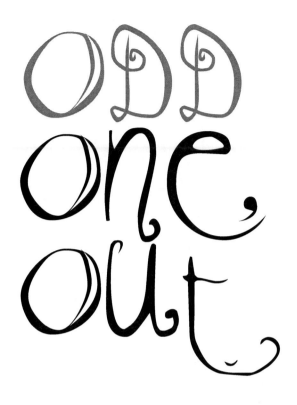

THE MAVERICK'S GUIDE
TO ADULT ADD

How to Be Happy and Successful by Breaking the Rules

JENNIFER KORETSKY

Odd One Out: The Maverick's Guide to Adult ADD

Copyright © 2007 by Jennifer Koretsky

The ideas and suggestions contained in this book are not intended as a substitute for consulting with your physician. All matters regarding your health require medical supervision. Neither the author nor the publisher shall be liable or responsible for any loss or damage allegedly arising from any information or suggestion in this book.

The names and identifying details of the client examples described in this book have been changed to preserve the confidentiality of the coaching relationship.

ISBN: 978-1-4276-2497-0

Library of Congress Control Number: TX 6-870-926

Cover design, layout and typesetting by Sarah Van Male, Cyanotype Book Architects.

Author photograph by Michael Polito, Michael Polito Photography.

Edited by Caille Howe, C.S. Howe Business Writing Services.

Published by Vervanté.

Printed in the United States of America

ADD Management Group, Inc.
P.O. Box 303
Plattekill, NY 12568
http://www.ADDmanagement.com

This book is dedicated to my partner, Erin.

Thank you for always believing in me,
supporting me, and—most of all—
for putting up with me.

ACKNOWLEDGEMENTS

Thank you to all of my clients. I won't list you here to respect your privacy, but know that whether we worked together for a short time or a long time, I learned as much from you as you did from me. I couldn't have written this book without you.

Thank you to my coaches: David Giwerc, Chris Barrow, and Andrea J. Lee. I learned more from the 3 of you than I did in all my years of formal education.

Thank you to my mental health support network past and present: Tatyana Timoff-Kissin, Adella Wasserstein, Julia Eilenberg, and Sil Reynolds.

Thank you to the Raise Your Game Master Mind Group: Chris Barrow, Jayme Broudy, Jamie Broughton, Paul Copcutt, Sandra de Freitas, Doug Emerson, Andrew Finkelstein, Stacey Hylen, and Sital Ruparelia. May we always have good coaching, great ideas, and fun times.

Thank you to my mother, Rita, for being a great role model and for unconditional love and support. And thanks for the all the funny stories I have to tell about you. You're truly an "odd one out" and you make me proud.

Thank you to my ADD-land colleagues for your friendship and support: Linda Anderson, Tom Dooley, Malka Engel, Blythe Grossberg, Terry Matlen, Tara McGillicuddy, Sondra Schiff, and Chris Speed.

Thank you to my ADD celebrities: Ned Hallow-

ell and Sari Solden. You inspired me to embrace
my maverick nature.

Thank you to all the wonderful people at
ADDA.

And finally, big thanks and lots of kisses to my
little babies, Punky and Rascal, for providing the
very best kind of distraction.

ATTENTION!

This is an ADD-friendly book. That means that you have permission to:

- Read the entire book in one sitting
- Take 6 months to read it
- Only read the chapters that interest you
- Mark up your book with notes and highlights
- Read and re-read until you get it
- Love it
- Hate it
- Take what you need and leave the rest

TABLE OF CONTENTS

mav·er·ick
(mav'er-ik, mav'rik)
Noun

One that refuses to abide by the dictates of
or resists adherence to a group; a dissenter. [1]

The odd one out. [2]

---

1 "maverick." The American Heritage® Dictionary
of the English Language, Fourth Edition. Houghton
Mifflin Company, 2004. 08 May. 2007. Available at:
http://dictionary.reference.com/browse/maverick.
2 Me.

Introduction

※

Embracing the Maverick

My name is Jennifer Koretsky, and I'm a maverick. I'm used to being the odd one out. I have adult ADD—*Attention Deficit/Hyperactivity Disorder*. I'm actually proud of that fact! I don't think that ADD is a bad thing. Sure, I have my share of challenges. But I think having ADD means that I have a lot of gifts and talents that many people only wish they possessed.

When you first get your ADD diagnosis, it's normal to be both relieved and disappointed. You're not crazy! Finally, there is an explanation as to why you do what you do. But it can also be disheartening. If you had only known sooner, imagine where you might be right now.

It's true. If you had some help and understanding along the way from those around you, you might be in a much different place. But that doesn't mean you're in a bad place right now. Your experiences in life—both good and bad—made you who you are. Your struggles have only made you stronger. **At this point in your life, you have a choice. You can choose to see your ADD as a disability, or a difference.** You can feel sorry for yourself, or you can embrace your differences and take pride in your maverick nature. One path leads to even more challenges and even lower self-esteem. The other leads to self-acceptance, improved self-esteem, happiness, and success.

Throughout this book, I'm going to reveal all my "secrets" and help you to view your ADD as an asset, too.

I'll be taking you through what I call **The 5 Essential Skills for Managing Adult ADD.** This is my roadmap for living successfully and happily. These are the skills that I live by, and the skills that I teach my clients in my work as an ADD Coach. They are designed to be simple guidelines you can follow to help you succeed in life while still being yourself.

Before getting started, I think you should know something about me and my journey. It's important to me that you understand where I'm coming from and why you can trust what you read in this book. So I'm going to tell you my story. I'll bet you can relate to a lot of it.

I was diagnosed with ADD, by accident, when I was 26. But first, let's back up. I grew up in a town in New York State, about 90 miles north of New York City. I hated it.

I did well in school, and I had friends. But I always felt like an outsider. I didn't really have a particular reason for feeling this way, I just did. I later found out that many ADDers felt like outsiders growing up.

More than anything, though, I was bored in my small town. As a teenager, I might get into a bar with a fake ID—if I was lucky. And yes, I used a fake ID all the time. I also drank and smoked pot. I rebelled here and there, probably out of boredom, but for the most part I was a good kid.

Most of my nights out consisted of the mall, McDonalds, a random party, or endless driving with friends. My town really had nothing to offer me, and I knew that after college I would be moving to a much more exciting place—New York City.

I had fun in college, but I could have had more fun. I actually enjoyed school when I could pick the subject matter that I was studying. I studied a lot and got good grades. In fact, most of my self-esteem came from those good grades. They were all I really had to feel good about. And if I had to do it all over again, I would have built my self-esteem, studied less, and had more fun.

Moving to the city after college was good for me. I enjoyed the freedom. Ever since I can remember, I have always been independent. I was "mature for my age," always looking to the next milestone. Wherever I was at, I was bored and ready to move on to new and exciting things.

And even in the city, **I got bored easily with**

the big things in my life—like my apartment. In 4 years I lived in 3 different apartments, finally buying an apartment when I was 25, where I ended up staying for almost 5 years—a record!

I also got bored with my jobs. If they weren't challenging, I found it difficult to get up in the morning. I worked for only 2 different companies before I started my coaching business, but I was constantly sending out my resume and going on job interviews, looking for something better. **It was almost like my mind couldn't sit still.** If I wasn't bored with my apartment, I was bored with my job. If I wasn't bored with my job, I was bored with who I was dating. I had a restless mind!

It was during this time that I decided to get psychotherapy. In addition to the family issues that we all have, there was one incident in particular that made me realize I needed some help and it was time to get therapy. This is the point where my life turned around. If you've ever attended one of my presentations, then you'll be familiar with the following anecdote.

THE SUBWAY INCIDENT

One morning I was on my way to work, riding a crowded New York City subway train. I was late, as usual. I had an early meeting that I still needed to prepare for. I was suffering from tremendous guilt, too, because I had just gotten a puppy, and she cried and whimpered whenever I left her. This was normal puppy behavior, but I still felt very bad! And to top it off, I was wet from the freezing rain I had to walk through to get to the subway—because even though I had taken out my umbrella and put it next to my bag, I had still forgotten to take it with me.

If all this wasn't bad enough, I was standing on the subway (getting a seat at rush hour was impossible) and I was next to some guy who kept stepping on my foot. Now, rush hour trains in New York City tend to get backed up. It's not uncommon to have your train move a few feet, stop short, and wait, over and over again. So if you aren't holding on, you'll lose your balance when the train stops and starts. And the guy next to me just didn't get that!

The first time he stepped on me, I huffed. You know, one of those deep sighs that communicates you're unhappy. The second time he stepped on me, I huffed *and* gave him a look. You know, one of those "if looks could kill" glances.

Remember, *I'm completely overwhelmed at this point.* I'm wet, I'm late for a meeting that I'm not prepared for, my train isn't going anywhere, I feel guilty for leaving my whimpering puppy, and this idiot keeps stepping on my foot. So the third time he did it, *I lost it.*

I yelled at him, I swore at him, and I nearly had a breakdown. It wasn't even 9:00 in the morning yet, and *my fuse was blown.* And the scary thing was that this wasn't even the first time that I completely lost it and exploded, unable to hold it together, before my day had even started.

From the outside looking in, I had a great life—I was a superstar in my company, a financial success, had a nice apartment, good friends, and a supportive family. **But I was constantly overwhelmed.**

I always felt like I was running behind on life. My apartment was never neat or clean enough. I didn't go to the grocery store or the laundromat often enough. I was late to my appointments. I looked around at everyone else and saw a city full of people who "had their shit together."

Yet, no matter how hard I worked and no matter how much I accomplished, I never felt like *I* had it together. I put so much pressure on myself, and I was always stressed out and overwhelmed. **Living life that way was so taxing, so stressful, that it didn't take much for me to completely fall apart.**

And that day, as I yelled and swore and nearly had a breakdown on a New York City subway train at 9:00 in the morning, I knew that something had to change.

GETTING MY DIAGNOSIS

I made the decision to get psychotherapy. My therapist was a wonderful woman. She never caught my ADD, but working with her changed my life. She introduced me to yoga and mediation; 2 things that helped me learn how to slow down that restless brain of mine.

She also helped me get over a lot of those "family issues" that we all have. And she helped me appreciate what I had, instead of constantly defaulting to boredom.

One day, however, I called her in a state of overwhelm. I don't remember what I was upset about, but I felt like I was losing it again. At that point she said to me, "You know, Jennifer, we've been working together for about a year now, and even though you've done some great work, you're still having more bad days than good. I think you might have dysthymia, a low level depression, and I'd like you to consider medication. I know a great psychiatrist that I can refer you to."

I was devastated. I felt betrayed. I thought that I had been doing really well. The breakdowns and blown fuses were happening less and less. I didn't understand why one little incident would indicate that I needed medication! **I didn't realize that most people don't constantly fight to ward off those internal breakdowns and blown fuses.**

I resisted calling the psychiatrist, but I eventually did. I explained to the doctor that lately I had been really stressed out. I would lose it over little things. I was bored at work and found myself daydreaming at meetings. I could pay attention if I was interested, but when management would go on and on about little financial details and procedural changes, I preferred to imagine what life would be like as a rock star. (I still do that every now and then.)

I also told her that I had "the grass is always greener syndrome," and that I always felt like there was a better job, or a better apartment waiting for me. I told her that I was annoyed with myself for not having a clean apartment, and because I ordered in all the time due to a lack of food in the fridge. I always intended to clean on Saturdays, but never felt like it once Saturday came around. Mondays were supposed to be my food shopping night, but most of the time I was too tired after work to bother going.

And I confessed that I had a hard time holding myself together. I told her about the subway incident and explained that these little meltdowns happened more than I cared to admit. I rarely took out my frustration on subway strangers, but I frequently felt overwhelmed to the point of bubbling over.

The more I talked, the more disheartened I became. "I hate living this way," I sighed.

She listened carefully. And then she said something that I will never forget. "Jennifer, I don't think you're depressed. I think you have Attention Deficit Disorder. ADD."

I nearly fell off the couch. *Clearly, this doctor was nuts.*

To me, ADD was something that made little kids annoying. Whenever I heard "ADD," I always thought about that little boy in my first grade class who couldn't sit still and be quiet. He would tap me on the shoulder to talk to me when I was taking a test or trying to pay attention. That surely wasn't me!

And I wasn't a kid, either. I was an adult! I might be in my 20s, but *I owned my apartment*, for goodness sake! ADD was for children, and I was no child.

"Um," I protested. "I don't think you understand. I was never hyperactive, and I'm not now. Quite the opposite! A lot of times I don't have the energy to do *anything!* And I was good in school, too! I loved school! When June came, I couldn't wait for September!

"And they love me at work!" I continued to protest. "I might get bored now and then, but I do a good job.

"And I can pay attention when I want to. I might daydream at work, but if I want to pay attention to you, I can! Like now, *you have my full attention!*" I insisted.

The doctor just nodded her head in agreement. She explained that ADD is often misunderstood. She said that the term "attention deficit" is misleading, because people with ADD don't really have an attention deficit, they have *attention inconsistencies*. But honestly, at that point, it didn't matter what she said to me. I didn't think there was any way in hell I had ADD.

She could sense my resistance, and she asked me to go buy a book called *Driven to Distraction: Recognizing and Coping with Attention Deficit Disorder from Childhood through Adulthood* by Drs. Ned Hallowell and John Ratey. We made an appointment for the next month.

It took me 3 weeks to buy that book. Not that I didn't have the opportunity to, I just didn't think there was any point in wasting the money on a book about a condition that I clearly didn't have. I finally caved, though, simply because I had an appointment with the doctor scheduled and I had promised I'd read the book. And when I finally did start to read it, I couldn't stop. By the third chapter, I was in tears. It was clear that I did, in fact, have ADD.

Driven to Distraction explained so many things about me that I always thought were character flaws. I learned that I really wasn't a horrible person who blew up at strangers for no good reason. **All my life, I had felt miserably overwhelmed and ready to blow at the slightest upset...but all my life I had done the best that I could with the knowledge and the tools that I had.**

A new world opened up to me just by reading about others who felt the same way that I did. And little did I know that *Driven to Distraction* was the beginning of so many great things to come for me.

I continued to see that psychiatrist, who wasn't crazy after all. She turned out to be a wonderful doctor and resource for me. It took a long time, but we found a psychostimulant medication that helped with my ADD and didn't have side effects. I also began taking medication for anxiety. Although my anxiety was never crippling, I had been going through life with a low level of anxiety that often had a hand in my becoming easily overwhelmed.

The combination of these 2 medications has done wonders for me. I have long since gotten over my fear and shame about taking medication. I'm a great person with a lot to offer, and the medication is merely a tool that helps me along the way.

The more I learned about ADD, the more I felt the pressure lifting. I wasn't the only one who felt overwhelmed and disorganized. I also wasn't the only one that drove myself to achieve more and more, despite all the stress and overwhelm.

I started to see that adults with ADD were something of an oddity in the world. **We didn't do things like everyone else, but we didn't need to beat ourselves up because of it.** I realized that I didn't need to be just like everyone else in order to be happy.

I let go of a lot of my own self-criticism. I started dropping off my laundry instead of stressing about when I would do it. And I got my groceries delivered, too. I even hired a cleaning person to come in every now and then! I was still late to work just about every day, but I felt like I had so much to offer that a couple of minutes here and there weren't such a big deal. Too bad the company that I worked for didn't agree!

The more I embraced myself as the person that I was and the person that I wanted to be, the more I realized that I didn't have to be stuck following the rules

that other people follow. I no longer wanted to define "having my shit together" in the same way that other people did. I no longer felt the need to be neat and organized and on time, *all the time.* I didn't want to follow the rules that didn't work for me. **I wanted to create my own rules in my own game, and play that game in a big way.** That meant being a maverick. It meant being the odd one out.

THE MAVERICK WITHIN

After this epiphany, it was immediately obvious that I would have to leave the corporate world. My corporate jobs were where most of my stress of "trying to fit in" came from.

My lateness was always noticed. My brilliant ideas were rarely noticed.

My difficulty following the pointless, bureaucratic rules was always noticed. My innovative systems for increased results weren't praised; they were viewed as unnecessary.

I was going home every night pissed off and drained. I didn't fit in. *And I didn't want to fit in.*

I started to think about how I might escape the corporate world. I resolved to ride it out a little while and be open to opportunities. I was surprisingly calm and patient about the process, and it worked.

A few months later, a colleague announced that he was leaving his job in the sales division to become a coach. We laughed at him. Personal and business coaching were fairly new at that point. Not many people in the general public understood what it was all about.

In the back of my head, however, I was remembering Ned Hallowell and John Ratey talking about coaching in *Driven to Distraction*. They suggested that ADDers could really benefit from a cheerleader who can hold them accountable. A light bulb appeared over my head.

That night I went home and began researching ADD coaching—for hours. And hours. I'm not sure I slept. I'll bet you know the feeling. Once I got this idea in my head, I was obsessed with it.

I talked to my psychiatrist and my therapist about the possibility of becoming an ADD coach and, to my surprise, they both thought it was a great idea. I was afraid they would doubt me, just as I doubted myself. After all, I had just learned about my own ADD fairly recently. I hadn't been working with my new ADD management systems for very long, and I still had things to learn. What right did I have to help other people when I was so new at this myself?

I didn't know it then, but I know now exactly why I had the right, *the obligation*, to help others. Yes, I had ADD all my life and didn't know it. In many ways the challenging aspects of ADD made my life difficult, disappointing, and incredibly stressful. But in many other ways, the positive attributes of ADD helped me to achieve great things in my life. To be proud of who I was. To be happy with myself and what I had to offer the world. I was succeeding in life, ADD and all.

I had a deep level of self-awareness, and I was always willing to learn and improve. **I had a special knack for using my ADD traits to my advantage.** And I did that by allowing myself to be the odd one out, even when it was really uncomfortable.

It became clear to me that if you treat ADD like a problem, it will become a problem.

If you treat it like a set of qualities and characteristics that help make you who you are, you can learn to manage the challenges and utilize the advantages.

I thrive outside of the mold. Most of the time, I *like* being the odd one out.

So with support from the people that I admired and trusted, I got my own coach, took a coach training course, and started coaching part time. Then in June of 2003, I held my breath and jumped: I quit my corporate job. I put myself in a "sink or swim" situation because I knew that was the only way I could make it work. I had something to prove—to my worried parents, my skeptical coworkers, and to some fellow coaches who insisted I couldn't make a living coaching full time. More importantly, I had something to prove to myself.

And here I am. I succeeded. And I did it on my terms.

I coach because I like working with adults

with ADD. I coach because I'm good at it. I coach because I've learned how to manage my own ADD and live out loud. I coach because it allows me to make my own rules. And I coach because I like mavericks. I want to give every adult with ADD the permission to make their own rules. I want to look around and see a world full of mavericks.

THE 5 ESSENTIAL SKILLS FOR MANAGING ADULT ADD

Breaking the rules can absolutely help you get ahead, but even mavericks need some structure. Having just a few, simple guidelines for living will allow you to be successful without compromising who you are. It helps to take your cues from the people who have already made their ADD work for them.

When I first began coaching, I started to notice something that I found peculiar. When I looked around at my clients, friends, and colleagues with adult ADD, I saw 2 groups of people: those who were successful, and those who struggled.

1. Successful ADDers
Successful ADDers have their challenges, but either learn to manage those challenges, or just accept them and move on. Their challenges don't stop them. This group isn't without problems, though. Many are their own worst enemies,

holding themselves to extremely high standards. But even though they might stress out some-times, these ADDers generally have what they want in life, and are always striving to reach the next level. These are people who absolutely have ADD, but just don't seem to fit into those ADD stereotypes. They are mavericks who embrace their differences.

2. Struggling ADDers
And then there are the adults with ADD who aren't so successful. They're not very happy. Their self-esteem is practically nonexistent. They never miss an opportunity to put themselves down. They struggle with extremely negative attitudes. They are always running late, and can't stay organized. They are stressed and overwhelmed almost all the time. They struggle to reach their goals for just a brief period of time before giving up all together. Which, of course, leads to even more self-esteem problems. They are more concerned about fitting in than they are about being happy.

Which group do you best fit into?

I consider myself to be in the first group. Sure, I had some problems with ADD and other things but, for the most part, I was successful. If I wanted something, I went after it. I got it. I felt good. There were other ADDers like me, but not very many. I was really curious about why this was.

So I started to take a look at that first group of

ADDers. I started with myself, and then I looked at my clients, friends and colleagues who were successful, and some famous ADDers, too.

I realized that we had something that other ADDers didn't. Sure we had our periods of struggle, but we bounced back from them because we had learned certain skills that helped us get ahead. These skills didn't necessarily come easily. In fact, many of them were difficult to learn. *But we learned them.*

And No matter how much you understand and practice a skill, you can always get better. The successful ADDers know this.

I determined, through my research, that there were **5 Essential Skills** that successful adults with ADD have mastered. To be a happy and successful ADDer, you have to know how to:

1. **Break the Cycle of Overwhelm**
2. **Work With Your ADD, Not Against It**
3. **ADDjust Your Attitude**
4. **Take Control of Your Space and Time**
5. **Live Out Loud**

I live these 5 skills every day of my life. That's what makes me a great ADD coach. I've "been there and done that" and I practice every strategy that I coach my clients on. When a client comes to me with a problem or challenge, I can always bring it back to one of these 5 skills. I'm going to show you how to do the same.

WHAT TO EXPECT

It's important to note that these skills will not "cure" or "fix" Attention Deficit/Hyperactivity Disorder. (And as you'll see, I truly believe that having ADD can be an asset in life.) This book is designed to help you increase your self-awareness, identify areas for growth, and build the ADD management skills that you may be lacking—without changing who you are.

It's also worth noting that coaching is part of a comprehensive ADD treatment plan. The skills and strategies contained in this book are not a substitute for medication, psychotherapy, or any other form of healthcare or treatment.

I know that learning these skills can sometimes be hard. I know that change doesn't come easily. But I also know that these skills work.

You can expect to have difficulties learning certain skills, and an easier time learning others. You can expect to have setbacks—we all do. And you can expect that you will not have mastered, or maybe even developed, these skills by the end of this book. If it were that easy, you'd already be managing your ADD. If it was that easy to change old habits and thought patterns, there would be no need for therapists, coaches, or self-help books. Life would be simple. And it would be boring.

My hope for you is that you begin to develop some of these skills in small steps, and some of them in giant leaps. Recognize that change requires time, energy, dedication, and *practice.*

I believe that true, lasting change happens in a 4-part process:

1. Education

It's information that inspires change. Becoming educated about ADD and the ways it can affect you is the first step to identifying changes that need to be made. This stage can last quite a long time before the next step is undertaken. Knowledge is like a seed and will grow in your mind all by itself. You're already on your way to change, just by reading this book.

2. Awareness

Self-awareness is key when making personal change. It's impossible to change that which you are not aware of. You have to practice self-awareness in all areas of life to determine what's working, and what isn't. You'll start to realize that certain behaviors and actions have propelled you forward, and others have held you back.

3. Reframing

It's important to realize that every person always does the best they can. No one purposefully underperforms, underachieves, or disappoints. When you give yourself enough credit to explore why you might do certain things the way you do, you can reframe your behaviors and actions with the understanding that they are there for a reason, and not because you are inadequate.

4. Action

Here's some great news: the action steps often happen all on their own! When you gain knowledge, practice awareness, and realize the positive reasons that change needs to take place, action will unconsciously follow. Of course, you can help it along. But don't be surprised if a year from now, or even a few weeks from now, you've made some major changes without even noticing that it was happening.

Change is something that we will practice our entire lives. Real, lasting change takes time, and can't be rushed. The important thing is that you've already begun the process.

I invite you to visit the *Odd One Out* website to access additional resources and materials that I've compiled just for readers. You can visit the Reader's Resources webpage at
www.odd-one-out.net/resources.html
at any time for more information and additional recommendations on the subject matter covered in this book.

Because these resources are just for *Odd One Out* readers, the webpage is not being made public. So be sure to type in the web address correctly to access the resources!

Note: Depending on your web browser, you may need to type
http://www.odd-one-out.net/resources.html
to access the page.

YOUR LIFE, YOUR RULES

When I first began seeing the therapist who I mentioned earlier, she invited me, and all her clients, to join her for a weekend trip to a yoga ashram in upstate New York. Many people don't realize that yoga is actually a religion and a way of life, not just a form of exercise. And this ashram that we visited was a religious retreat where yoga practitioners and swamis lived. Knowing I wasn't religious, my therapist told me, "Take what you want from the experience and leave the rest."

My first ashram trip was a difficult one. The food was a little too healthy for me and although the center was a beautiful mountain retreat, I was somewhat antsy. Plus, yogis get up at the crack of dawn to do yoga and meditate! It wasn't easy, but I went with the flow. It was relaxing and peaceful, and I was in serious need of some stress relief.

On the first evening of my retreat, however, something strange happened. I had dinner with the group and proceeded to *satsang*, which was described to me as meditation followed by a group discussion with one of the swamis. To my surprise, after our meditation, people began passing out small musical instruments, like drums and tambourines. Before I knew it, the whole group was chanting and playing instruments. I looked around and freaked out. *My therapist is in a cult!* I screamed silently. *I've been recruited to a religious cult by my therapist!*

When I later confronted her about my fears,

she calmly answered, "I told you to take what you want and leave the rest. You are free to join in the activities, or just relax."

Oh.

I have since grown to love ashram retreats— even satsang. There is actually something very calming about chanting in a group and gently banging on an instrument. I don't even know what I'm saying as I chant, and it doesn't matter. It helps me feel peaceful and centered.

So here's my advice to you, based on my own life lesson from the ashram experience: **take what you want from this book and leave the rest.**

I'm going to tell you all about **The 5 Essential Skills for Managing Adult ADD**. While I do believe that these skills are absolutely necessary for all adults with ADD, I'm not as concerned about how you master them. It doesn't matter *how* you develop the skills, as long as you *do* develop them.

I'm going to offer you many strategies, tools, and suggestions. Some will appeal to you and some won't. That's okay. Take what you want and leave the rest.

Feel free to use the suggestions that work for you and ignore the ones that don't. Take the ideas and strategies that don't fit perfectly, and adjust them as you like.

I'll offer the guidelines, and you make the rules. Between the 2 of us, you'll get what you need to embrace your own maverick nature, and live happily and successfully.

Are you ready to stop trying to fit in? Are you ready to embrace being the odd one out? Are you ready to proudly label yourself a maverick?

Then let's get started!

Chapter 1

※

Break the Cycle
of Overwhelm

OVERWHELM: THE COMMON DENOMINATOR

"I'm just so overwhelmed... I don't even know where to begin."

This is what many of my coaching clients tell me during our very first conversation. It's a state of being that I am all too familiar with.

Adult ADD is more than distractibility, impulsivity, and inattention. While these *are* the 3 symptoms we hear about most often, ADD affects us all in different ways. You may or may not see your biggest challenges in these 3 symptoms. But I believe that there is one thing that we all do have in common, and that is *we become easily overwhelmed with everyday life.*

Our internal filters don't work the same way that other people's do, and we end up focusing our awareness on too many things at one time. What's worse is that some of the things we are paying attention to aren't even relevant in the present! Sometimes we don't even *care* about what we're paying attention to.

When your focus is on so many things at once, no matter what actually gets done, there's always much more waiting for your attention. There is so much to do at home, at work, at school, or wherever, that it feels like you just can't possibly do it all. **You feel like you're always running so far behind that you'll never catch up.**

This is the world of adult ADD.

Because of this, many of us end up feeling like we must move as fast as possible in order to hold everything together. Sometimes, the very thought of everything that needs to be held together is so overwhelming that we lose our motivation to make progress.

It doesn't take much for you to get overwhelmed, does it? You might have a lot going on in your life and find yourself holding it all together really well, and then something completely insignificant will throw you into overwhelm. Walking into a cluttered room can do it. Trying to get through your email Inbox can do it. Getting a new assignment at work or at school can do it. Sometimes, the smallest things can throw you completely off track.

That uncomfortable yet familiar state of overwhelm sets in, and you become frantic. You might shift into "high" speed, working on overdrive to get it all done, feeling stressed the whole time. And at the end of the day, it feels like you're no further along than when you started. How frustrating!

Or, you may have the opposite reaction to overwhelm. It may have you feeling depressed and confused, with no idea where to start. You find yourself procrastinating all day. You're painfully aware of what you need to do, but just can't muster up the motivation.

Have you ever sat on the couch, watching TV, eating ice cream, and metaphorically kicking yourself for not getting off your butt to clean the house like you promised yourself you would?

Either way, the result is that you feel guilty, lazy, disorganized, and stressed out because you're just not being productive. Those feelings often lead to beating yourself up, because it "shouldn't be this hard." So now you add low self-esteem to this already awful mix of feelings and that, in turn, adds to the overwhelm!

Once you enter the state of overwhelm, it's very difficult to break out of it. In fact, the state of overwhelm usually ends with a period of absolute burnout, in which you may find yourself losing your temper, shutting down, or even getting sick.

Now, here's the worst part: even after the burnout period, you know that it probably won't be long until you go into overwhelm again.

It's not your fault. If you knew how to stop this cycle, you would have done it by now. Just because you haven't figured it out yet doesn't mean that there isn't hope! Getting out of overwhelm won't just help you feel more relaxed and together, it will allow you the time and energy you need to build other ADD management skills. Plus, it will free up some of your time to enjoy life, too!

THE GOLDEN RULE OF ADD MANAGEMENT

Arguably, the most important piece in learning how to break the cycle of overwhelm is remembering what I call 'The Golden Rule of ADD Management:' **Your ADD challenges directly correlate to your stress levels.**

The more stressed out you are, the more your ADD will challenge you and present problems.

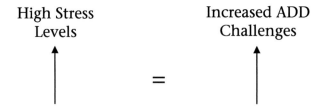

Conversely, when you are calm, centered, and relaxed, your ADD will be much more manageable, and can even be used to your advantage.

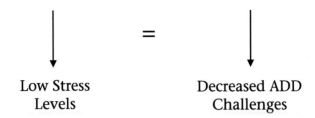

Low Stress
Levels

Decreased ADD
Challenges

Have you ever noticed that when you're stressed out, it's more difficult to get to your appointments on time? You tend to forget more things, too—like where you put the keys—when you're *already* running late for that appointment.

During times like these, every traffic light you approach turns red, you're guaranteed to spill your drink, and you'll rush into your appointment in a discombobulated frenzy.

Admittedly, there is some humor in this when you remember these experiences from a distance. In the moment, however, it's awful.

The more stressed out you are, the more your ADD affects you in negative ways. And the more your ADD affects you in negative ways, the more stressed out you become. What a vicious cycle! And we all get caught up in it.

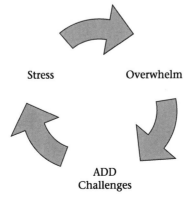

Stress   Overwhelm

ADD
Challenges

When you have adult ADD, stress very quickly becomes absolute and total overwhelm. Once overwhelm sets in, you become easily distractible and forgetful. You lose track of time. You feel disorganized. It affects every little thing you do.

It's impossible to learn how to manage your ADD without learning how to manage your stress.

SLOW DOWN TO SPEED UP

The "speedy" feeling that we experience in times of overwhelm can be mental and/or physical. If you're in a "high gear" state then you feel both mentally and physically hyperactive. If you're stuck on the couch procrastinating, your mind is still racing.

In the moment, the speediness feels appropriate. Either you have to move quicker to get things done, or you have to pressure yourself to get things done. But the truth is that you are simply not efficient in that speedy, frantic state. It causes chaos. How can you be productive in the middle of chaos? It just doesn't work.

You have to give yourself permission to take the time to step back from all the stress, drop your to-do's, and recharge. *You have to slow down.* While some people need to go into high gear to break out of overwhelm, this doesn't work for adults with ADD because it provides only a temporary fix that leads to burnout. Stepping back from the speediness is exactly what you need to do to stop it.

ADDers often resist the idea of slowing down. When there is always so much on your mind that needs attending to, the idea of slowing down seems counterintuitive. However, I think that most of us can agree that constantly feeling like you're operating on high speed is exhausting. In this state of mind, you spend so much energy trying to hold it all together that you no longer have the energy—or time—to do the things in life that you actually enjoy. The maverick in you wants to emerge, but gets crushed by the weight of chaos and overwhelm.

It's nearly impossible to slow down if you don't have self-awareness. Being able to identify where and when you are becoming overwhelmed is the first step to slowing down. It sounds simple, and it is. We often don't realize that we're on high speed until we already feel overwhelmed and disorganized. Building your awareness of these tendencies is the first and biggest step towards stopping them!

Once you have increased your awareness of your speedy tendencies in day-to-day life, you can begin to develop strategies that will help you slow down and feel less overwhelmed. The strategies that you put into place will be based on your specific personality and your specific needs. The concept of "slowing down" will be applied differently for everyone. **It's important to ex-**

periment with different strategies to find out which ones work for you. You make the rules.

For some, weekly time-outs for fun or relaxation will be helpful. For others, one or more small chunks of downtime each day will be necessary to avoid overwhelm.

I recommend that all ADDers spend some time each day slowing down. If this is hard for you, start with a small amount of time, and build up. Even 5 minutes of downtime each day will make a big difference.

WAYS TO SLOW DOWN

There are lots of ways that you can choose to slow down. But first, let's get really clear about what it means to slow down.

Slowing down doesn't mean stopping. Rather, **slowing down is about removing yourself from stressful situations so that you can relax and de-stress**.

Some good ways to slow down are:

- Taking a walk
- Journaling
- Meditating
- Listening to music
- Practicing yoga
- Playing with kids
- Spending time with pets

- Crafting (knitting, wood working, scrap booking, etc.)
- Being artistic (singing, painting, writing, dancing, etc.)
- Practicing a hobby
- Exercising
- Taking a drive
- Going out for a meal
- Going out with friends
- Reading for pleasure (as opposed to reading for school or work)
- Taking a nap
- Watching TV

You may want to use the margins to jot down any other ideas you have to slow down.

When you choose an activity to help you slow down, make sure it's not something that you can get "sucked into." For example, watching TV can help you slow down only if you can walk away from it. If you find yourself getting sucked into movies or shows, or unable to turn the TV off, then it's not a good method of slowing down. The time you waste will only make you feel worse.

That's not to say that TV is a bad thing or that you should never watch it. I love TV. There are plenty of shows that I simply *have* to watch every week, and I will plan my life around them! But TV shouldn't be used as a method of slowing down if you, like me, have a tendency to get wrapped up in it.

I'm a reality TV junkie. But reality TV is full of

some stressful things, like intense conflict, races to the finish, and strategies for survival. All of this stuff gets my brain going! It's great to watch, but too stimulating to use as a method of slowing down.

Something that you won't find on the list of ways to slow down is anything related to computers. **The Internet, email and computer games are like quicksand for ADDers!** You may tell yourself that you'll only be on the computer for a few minutes but, before you know it, you're hunched over the keyboard with stiff muscles and sore eyes, telling yourself "just 2 more minutes."

I've often said that you know you have ADD if you've ever been on the computer at 3:00 a.m. researching *exactly* how potatoes grow in Idaho… only to find that you could care less the following day. All you know is that a question popped into your head in the middle of the night and you felt compelled to find the answer immediately.

The point is that computers are easy to hyper-focus on and get caught up in; and therefore, they are *not* a good method of slowing down.

You know you've got yourself a good slowing down activity when you find that it helps you escape your day and forget about your stress for a little while. Some people will find that exercise helps them do this; while others will find that they need a very quiet and calm activity with no distractions, like meditation. Whatever works for you is what you should stick with!

Take some time to experiment with different activities until you find a few that work for you. Stay flexible. The goal is merely to let your stress go and relax for a short period of time each day.

RECHARGE YOUR BATTERIES

Have you ever been walking or exercising with an mp3 player (or walkman, or radio) and the batteries run out? What happens?

Well, if you're like me, the first thing you do is play with the batteries! *Hmmm...what if I take them out and switch their positions?* It might work for 2 minutes, but that's it. The batteries are simply out of energy and there is nothing you can do about it.

Did you know that this can happen to you, too?

Adults with ADD have a low tolerance for frustration. We also have a difficult time regulating our energy levels. So if you have a rough day at work, come home to find a sink full of dishes when you left it clean, and discover that your brand new shirt somehow managed to get badly stained, you're likely to find yourself blowing a fuse.

Blowing a fuse isn't about losing your temper, although that might happen. When an ADDer blows a fuse, it means that your energy has been zapped. You feel like you just can't handle anything else. The juice in your batteries is gone and you're done!

This is the perfect time to slow down. Don't succumb to the stress, just step back from it. Take an hour out to slow down, or take the rest of the day if you feel you need it. The problems aren't going to go away on their own. You'll have to deal with them eventually. Would you rather do so feeling calm and centered, or frantic and spent?

Let's explore this concept with another metaphor: filling your car with gas. I live in "the country." The dry cleaners are close to home, about 2 miles away. The nearest supermarket is 8 miles away. My bank is 10 miles away. And the farm where I like to buy organic meats and produce is 30 miles away.

Now, I have a bad habit of letting the gas tank in my car get pretty low before filling it. In fact, that little yellow light often comes on letting me know that I need gas. (Please, don't mention this to my mother. There are few things you could do to upset her more than to let your gas tank get below ¼ full. It's right up there with felony crime.)

So let's use this setup as our example. I need to visit all 4 places today, and my plan is to go to the bank first, then the grocery store, and then the farm, so that my fresh food has the shortest amount of time in the car. I'll stop at the cleaners last, because it's so close to home. It's a beautiful summer day and I'm in a great mood!

Now let's say that when I get in the car and prepare to run my errands, I notice that I have only ¼ tank of gas. *No biggie*, I think to myself, *I'll get gas on the way.*

I drive to the bank with no problem. It's on the way to the grocery store, so that makes life easier. I plan to stop for gas, but a good song comes on the radio and I get distracted. *No problem,* I think, *I'll get it on the way to the farm.*

I do what I need to at the bank and the grocery store, and I'm off to the farm. It's a long drive, but who cares! I have the radio on and I love driving. Just have to remember to fill the tank. It's starting to get low...

I pass a gas station on the way to the farm, but I can't believe how high the gas prices are! *The way home is a little more remote, so the gas stations will be cheaper. I'll wait,* I tell myself.

I go to the farm, chat with the farmer, get what I need, and get in the car. Wow! The little gas light is on already! I wasn't expecting that. Okay, gas is now a priority.

As I drive a lot of country back roads on my route home, I remember that there actually aren't any gas stations until I get much closer to home. *Uh-oh.*

The inevitable happens: I run out of gas. My car has run out of the fuel that it needs to operate properly. As a result, and a consequence, I am not able to finish running my errands. A large amount of my fresh food will probably expire in the hot car. I won't make it to the dry cleaners before closing. Not to mention the fact that I have to call for road service, and pay a lot of money for that road service. Plus, this inconvenience has me completely stressed out. What had been a good day has now turned into an awful one.

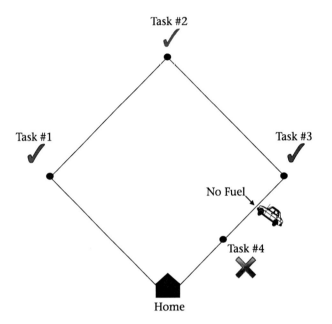

What did I do wrong? It's obvious, isn't it? I needed to stop for gas before I ran all my errands! If I had only taken the time to put a little gas in my tank, I wouldn't have all these problems.

Our bodies and minds are just like the gas tanks in our cars. If you don't stop to refuel them, they will run out of energy.

And when you have adult ADD, chances are that you have a smaller gas tank than most people. This is our "low tolerance for frustration" and our "difficulty regulating energy and alertness." Recharging is all about making sure that you don't run out of gas. It's about taking time out to relax and de-stress, so that you can handle the challenges that come your way.

Recharging for you may mean doing your slow-down activities midday. Or it may mean taking a walk on your lunch hour. It may also be as simple as taking several deep breaths throughout the day or reminding yourself to breathe when someone pisses you off. It's all about keeping your stress levels down.

These recharging breaks aren't a luxury. They are a necessity. It's not enough to say, "I'll recharge when I'm done with this or that," or "I'll recharge later." If you keep putting off that stop at the gas station, you'll run out of fuel.

This is actually a very simple and extremely helpful change that you can make in your life, and yet I frequently hear objections. The most popular one goes something like this: "But my best friend has it all together. She's married, has 2 kids, works, paints in her spare time, and is on the city council. She never slows down."

My response to that is "Yes...and? Don't make me say it. If your friend jumped off a bridge, would you feel like you were supposed to jump, too?"

Adults with ADD *need* this time to recharge and refuel. We're easily overwhelmed, easily frustrated, and have the propensity to burn out. Recharging is how you avoid that.

If it puts an extra step in your day, big deal. If it makes you the odd one out, who cares? Would you rather be calm and relaxed in between periods of recharging, or would you rather be miserable, stressed, and burnt out all the time?

Mavericks understand that the path to happiness and success requires frequent recharging. You don't get far when you're always burning out.

PUT ON YOUR OXYGEN MASK FIRST

I know you've probably heard this metaphor before, but I think it's worth reviewing. When you travel by plane, the flight attendants always do their safety spiel and include instructions on what to do if the cabin loses pressure and the oxygen masks drop down. **They tell you to make sure that you put on and secure your own mask first, before helping the person next to you.**

I've flown many times, and I have never once heard a flight attendant mention any exception to this rule. It doesn't matter if the person sitting next to you is your 2-year-old child, your 90-year-old mother, or a random stranger. You must put on your mask first!

The reason for this is really quite simple. If you try to help someone else fasten their mask first, you'll run out of air. And you can't help that person next to you—kid, mother, or stranger—if you can't breathe. If you do, you sacrifice yourself to save that person, and it's unnecessary. It doesn't take a lot of time to put on your mask first. You can take the time to make sure that you can breathe, and then help the other people around you. It's not selfish; it's practical.

This metaphor goes way beyond airplanes. It applies to your life.

Anna's Story

Anna was diagnosed with ADD in her late 30s. She sought treatment for postpartum depression and discovered that she had ADD as well. At the time, Anna was caving under all her responsibilities. She had a new daughter, a husband, a house, a business, and a large extended family that demanded a lot from her. One day, her brain just shut down.

Anna was raised in a big family and was taught from very early on that you always put your family first. Anna's family had no boundaries, and therefore Anna had no boundaries.

Like many of her brothers and sisters, and even her mother, Anna was a businesswoman. Arguably, she was the best businessperson in her family! Her family saw her as very successful, and expected her to take care of them. They came to her for everything from errands to money to help in their own businesses.

Being a people pleaser, and fearing the repercussions of saying no, Anna did what was asked of her. She felt like she was on a motor, going and doing for everyone else, even though she just had a baby! And yet, even though she did her best to take care of everyone else, she often couldn't follow through on her promises because she was so overwhelmed. This often left her family feeling angry with her.

Two things really helped Anna turn things around: medication and joining my group coaching program. The medication helped her focus and see things more clearly, while the coaching helped her see that she was becoming overwhelmed because she had no boundaries. She realized that she was helping everyone else, and no one was helping her. She was suffering, and so was her business.

Anna became the odd one out in her family and began putting up boundaries. She put herself first and made more time for her husband and daughter. Her clients came next. And if the family wanted Anna's consulting expertise in their businesses, then they would have to pay for her time, just like any other client.

Taking it even further, Anna began insisting on contracts for the work she did on family businesses. This way, the services she was expected to provide, along with the fee she was promised, would be clear to all. She was still helping her family, but it was no longer at her own expense.

When she first started saying no and putting up these boundaries, her family did not react well. They were used to the Anna who always said yes! But she didn't back down, and over time gained her family's respect.

The changes that she made influenced the whole family. She showed them that it's possible to love and care for your family without sacrificing yourself. Her relationships with her family have greatly improved.

More importantly, Anna no longer feels overwhelmed all the time! Putting herself first allowed her to move forward in all aspects of her life.

Many ADDers have difficulty getting their needs met. Our high level of compassion often has us worrying about others before ourselves. Sometimes, this is necessary. Your kids need to eat even if you're tired, your sick parent may need to go to the doctor even though you have to work, and your boss may need that report even though you are stressed to the max. Sometimes, this is just life, and we have to deal with it.

However, many adults with ADD feel that it is their responsibility to care *extensively* for others, even when it's clear that they are taking on unnecessary responsibilities.

In an effort to fit in and look like we have it all together, we end up going the extra mile for other people more often than we need to—certainly more often than we're asked to—and sometimes compromise our own needs in the process.

Think about all the people in your life whom you put before yourself. This might include your kids, your parents, your siblings, your pets, your friends, your boss, your coworkers, your neighbors, and others. How many people are you going short of breath for as you meet their needs before your own?

With all this time and energy spent caring for others, we tend to have less time to meet our own needs. What many adults with ADD don't realize is that **we are much less useful to those around**

us when our own needs are not being met. When you give and give and give of yourself, there is less *quality you* to go around. When you take care of yourself and get your own needs met, you operate from a place where you have much more to give to those around you.

Mavericks know that putting themselves first may mean a little less time with those they love. But mavericks also know that getting their needs met first ensures that the time they do spend with loved ones is much happier and more fulfilling for everyone.

SELF-CARE: POPPING THE BUBBLE BATH THEORY

Have you ever read a magazine article on self-care that instructs you to be good to yourself by taking a hot bath? Did you actually take a bath after reading that article, or did you roll your eyes?

Don't get me wrong; I love baths. Bubble baths are even better. Bubble baths in my whirlpool tub are wonderful. In fact, give me a hot tub with some candles and aromatherapy and I'm in relaxation heaven!

Baths are an excellent way to slow down and recharge. But when it comes to self-care for adults with ADD, there is a lot more to consider than bubble baths.

The primary elements of self-care are the ones we're most familiar with: eating properly, getting plenty of sleep, and exercising on a regular basis. I think we can all agree that when these 3 things are working for you, you *feel* better. There are a couple of other considerations that I'd add to this list, as well. The following are what I consider to be the top 5 guidelines for practicing excellent self-care.

1. Nourish Yourself

You have no doubt heard rumors that excess sugar causes ADD, but there has been no scientific evidence to date that backs this up. However, if you pay close attention to what you eat, I think you'll find that the foods you consume have a big effect on your ability to manage your ADD.

Take refined sugars and simple carbohydrates, for example. Refined sugars are all sugars that are not in their naturally occurring form. Carbohydrates in their naturally occurring forms are foods like fruits, vegetables, and whole grains. We find refined sugars in processed foods like cookies, cakes, jams, and even fast food.

Refined carbohydrates are "whites": white bread, white rice, and white pasta. Wheat, rice, and other grains are not found in nature in this white form. Most people eat refined carbohydrates that have been stripped of their fiber and naturally occurring vitamins and nutrients. These foods are often bleached, too. They may then be enriched with the vitamins they were originally stripped of, but the end result is a product that has been highly processed and breaks down into sugar when digested.

The problem with refined sugars and carbohydrates is that they cause a spike in your blood sugar, which causes a spike in your energy. But this energy burst doesn't last long before there is a drop in your blood sugar, and that causes a drop in your energy.

If you start your day off with some sugary cereal, you will get a burst of energy, but you will soon find yourself crashing, and craving more sugar and carbs. And thus the cycle continues—all day long your energy is spiking and dropping. You're feeling sluggish and tired from trying to keep up. Clearly, with all this stress on your physical body, it's going to be more difficult to manage your ADD.

And it's not just sugar and refined carbs that cause this cycle. Caffeine and nicotine have similar effects on the body. They screw up your blood sugar and your brain chemicals.

The experts that I listen to and agree with suggest eating *whole and real foods*, like fruits, vegetables, and whole grains. These are "good carbs." Some examples of whole grains are brown rice, corn, quinoa, millet, steel cut oats, amaranth and whole wheat. Take a trip to the "natural and organic" section of your grocery store, or to your local health food store, for a selection of whole grains that are easy to cook, taste great, and are absorbed slowly into your blood stream, which means they produce a slow, steady stream of energy.

There are some additional ways to ensure that your energy levels remain consistent throughout the day. One way is to eat protein with every meal, which can be in the form of meat, fish, fowl, dairy, nuts, beans, and legumes. (Experts tend to disagree on whether or not dairy is the best form of protein. All I know is that I love my milk, cheese, and yogurt. And ice cream. But pretend I didn't mention the ice cream part. I prefer milk and dairy from grass-fed cows, which is much more nutritious than industrial, mainstream dairy products.)

It's also important to eat when you're hungry. A small, balanced snack in response to hunger, like fresh fruit and nuts, will ensure that your blood sugar levels remain steady.

I'd be a hypocrite if I tried to pretend that I eat a perfectly balanced diet. Food is hard for many ADDers. There has even been some research on the prevalence of obesity in ADDers.

If you're not ready to make huge changes in your diet right now, I understand. It's not easy. So here is the gist of what you need to know: **The more you eat nutritious, whole foods, the better you will feel. The better you feel, the easier it is to manage your ADD.**

I slip up often. But instead of beating myself up about it, I get back on track as soon as possible, because I know that I always feel better when I eat nutritiously.

If you'd like more resources on good nutrition, and the relationship between obesity and ADD, visit the Odd One Out Reader's Resources webpage at **www.odd-one-out.net/resources.html**

2. Get Out Of Your Head and Into Your Body
Building on the principle that the better you feel the easier it is to manage your ADD, let's take a look at exercise.

I love and hate exercise at the same time. I love the way it makes me feel afterward. But I often hate doing it.

Exercise has so many benefits. It helps reduce stress, speeds up metabolism, makes your heart stronger, increases flexibility, increases oxygen to the cells in your body, and balances brain chemicals. We are all well versed in the health benefits of exercise. But what about the practical benefits?

Think about it for a moment...don't you *feel better* when you exercise regularly? In fact, when you stop exercising and then start up again, don't you wonder why you ever stopped in the first place?

Practically speaking, exercise feels good. It increases energy and focus, and helps you sleep better. It decreases your stress and tension levels. It gives you the opportunity to stop thinking so much, and move your body. You feel more balanced and in control. So of course, when you are exercising regularly, you feel better and, once again, it becomes much easier to manage your ADD.

There are lots of different ways to exercise, but the form that seems to be most beneficial for ADDers is aerobic exercise. This is the type of exercise that gets your heart going and makes you sweat! Power walking, jogging, running, biking, aerobics, racquetball, and many other sports and activities are aerobic exercise. It may be tough to do, but it feels so good afterwards!

Personally, I hate exercise when it involves being in a certain place at a certain time. I don't like the gym and I don't like group sports. I'd rather take my dogs for a moderate hike or work up a sweat doing yard work.

If you already do a fair amount of aerobic exercise, then good for you! Many ADDers I know find that aerobic exercise helps them manage ADD better than medication.

If you're not currently exercising, try to think about adding in some physical activity that you personally find fun and fulfilling. You are not confined to the gym for your exercise! This is one area in which it's really easy to embrace your maverick nature and use it to your benefit. Identify the forms of physical activity that make you happy, and then allow yourself to enjoy them.

I once had a client who enjoyed canoeing, but rarely allowed himself to spend the afternoon on the lake because there were always too many other things he had to do. When I pointed out that canoeing is exercise, it became easier for him to justify the time and schedule it in. It no longer seemed like procrastination or avoidance, it was self-care in the form of exercise.

Be sure to speak with your doctor before starting an exercise program. You absolutely want to make sure that your health is good before you begin exercising. If it turns out that you do have some problems to look out for, your doctor can work with you to find an appropriate exercise program that will be healthy and enjoyable.

The important thing to remember is that you'll benefit from any activity that takes you out of your head and brings you into your body.

3. Make Sleep a Priority

Sleeping problems are very common for adults with ADD. Many of us stay up later than we want to, have trouble falling asleep, have a hard time getting up in the morning, and feel sluggish throughout the day. Unfortunately, it takes some effort for many of us to regulate our sleep patterns.

We all know that to ensure we get proper sleep, we're *supposed* to go to bed and wake up at the same times each day. This is a great idea, but it's easier said than done!

If you don't sleep during the night, it's incredibly difficult to get up in the morning. So let's approach this subject a little backwards—starting with bedtime.

One of the problems ADDers face when trying to go to bed is that we get a "second wind." I'm guilty of this sometimes, but it used to be a lot worse! In the past, it was not uncommon for me to feel tired all evening, and then at about 10:00 p.m. feel wired. I would suddenly want to clean, organize, read, pick up old projects, exercise, and do anything and everything else that required a lot of energy.

The result was that I would feed that second wind, rile myself up, and be too wired to fall asleep. My brain was awake, even though my body was tired. And this always led to racing thoughts that would take over and run away with themselves, keeping me up even longer. When the ADD mind tries to be quiet, anxiety and worry often creep in. And once there, they tend to take over. Does this scenario sound familiar to you?

Most of my clients experience very similar challenges. I estimate that only about 10% of my clients go to bed easily, sleep well, and wake up feeling refreshed in the morning.

If you have a lifestyle that allows you to set your sleep schedule according to your own bio-rhythms, then good for you! As a maverick, you can give yourself permission to go with it as long as it works for you.

Many of us don't have that luxury, however, and are forced to find a compromise between our own biorhythms and the schedule that the rest of the world operates on.

The key to solving this problem is to go to bed feeling physically and mentally tired, instead of wired. In order to do this, you've got to cut out all the things that stimulate your mind a couple of hours before bedtime. This allows both your body and your mind to shut down before you get in bed.

This means that, depending on what stimulates you, you may have to cut out TV, reading, phone calls, and—no doubt about it, the computer—a couple of hours before you go to bed.

I know, you're probably gasping for breath right now. Turn off the TV? Put down the book? *Turn off the computer?*

Yes, turn off that computer! TV and reading...well, that depends. The computer—with email and Internet and games—is sure to wake you right up and stimulate your brain, meaning it will take you a lot longer to fall asleep once that computer is turned off.

You may find, however, that reading relaxes you and makes you sleepy. If that's the case, then reading is a good pre-bedtime activity for you! But be careful not to pick up a book that is a "page turner." You know, the kind that has you saying, "Just one more chapter!" at the end of *every* chapter.

And you may find that TV also helps you relax. If so, that's great! But beware—if you find yourself flipping channels late at night instead of turning the TV off at a pre-determined time, then that TV is sucking you in and stimulating your brain!

I'll admit this happens to me all the time. I can plan on watching a half-hour sitcom, but rarely ever turn the TV off afterwards. What happens is that I catch a quick glimpse of the next show, and then I just *have* to find out what happens! I even do it with old reruns, like *The Brady Bunch*. I remember the episode, and I *know* that Greg is going to get in trouble for not driving carefully, yet I can't seem to tear myself away.

Or, I know that I need to go to sleep, but I'll

flip through the 10 different HBO channels that I have to find a good movie, which will keep me up another hour and a half. Even though I want to turn that TV off, I somehow feel unable to do so.

So the solution, for me, is to not turn the TV on to begin with. It's just too stimulating for me to watch right before bed.

It's important to pay attention to what stimulates *you*, and stay away from those activities for an hour or 2 before bed. Give your body and mind the opportunity to shut down by doing other things that don't stimulate you—like taking a bath, meditating, or listening to soft music—and you'll find that it's much easier to fall asleep once you get into bed.

In the morning, do whatever it takes to get out of bed. If you have trouble waking up in the morning, you know by now that your alarm clock is nothing more than an annoyance that you can shut up for 9 minutes before fighting with it again.

Instead of relying on your alarm clock alone, try engaging your senses. Leave the curtains open before bed so the sun comes in during the morning. Set a stereo in another room to go off when you need to get up. Set up an air freshener or aromatherapy diffuser to turn on around the same time. Don't just try to wake up your body, wake up your mind by activating your senses.

In the same way that your mind needs to wind down at night, it also needs to wind up in the morning.

4. Like, Respect, and Trust Your Doctors

Many adults with ADD largely ignore one very important factor in self-care: health care providers.

Whether you're looking for a dentist or a general practitioner, it's tough to find good doctors today. Very few actually take the time to get to know you and develop a personal relationship with you. And (in the United States, at least) when you find a good one who does go out of their way to provide you with top-notch care, they usually don't take your insurance!

If you walk out of your doctor's office—*any* doctor's office—grumbling about what a jerk they are, then it is *not okay* to continue seeing them.

When you choose a doctor, you put your health in their hands. You trust them to determine if there are any problems that need to be addressed, and to help you take preventative measures for illnesses and diseases that you may be at risk for. **Never trust your care to someone who doesn't answer your questions or take your concerns seriously.**

While this makes sense on paper, it becomes a problem for many adults with ADD because finding good doctors requires a lot of time and effort. It's often easier to go to the doctor who is close by, or the doctor who takes your insurance, because you just don't feel like going through the process of looking for a new one. However, finding good doctors is an investment in yourself and your health.

The first and easiest thing you can do to find a good doctor is to ask around. Ask your friends, family, and neighbors who they recommend. This cuts down on a lot of research time, and if a doctor gets along well with someone whom you get along well with, then chances are you may be a good fit!

You can also check your health insurance provider's directory. If you find someone that looks good, try Googling their name. See what you can find out about that doctor online. Do they have a website or an online profile? Perhaps they have published a paper or appeared in an article. Or, if you're really lucky, you may come across a patient rating of the doctor! These are all great ways to get a sense of the doctor and their personality before you commit to a visit.

Lastly, try, try again. If you visit a doctor that you don't gel with, don't be afraid to stop seeing them, and see someone else, instead. Mavericks identify what they want and then go for it. A little extra effort isn't enough to stop them. Sure, all of these strategies can be time consuming and frustrating, but isn't your health worth it?

And by the way, everything said above applies to therapists, counselors, and coaches, too!

If You Are Taking Medication...

In the United States, most insurance companies reimburse health care providers so little that they are forced to see 4–5 patients an hour just to make a living. This is unfortunate. And it's particularly dangerous when a healthcare provider who sees you for 10 minutes a visit is your psychiatrist, or other doctor prescribing your ADD medication!

I always recommend that my clients see a psychiatrist for their ADD medication. And, due to the current state of the U.S. health insurance industry, it's not uncommon for a psychiatrist to stop taking insurance once they have established a practice.

But it's important to see a good psychiatrist that you like, respect, and trust *anyway,* even if it means that you pay more for your healthcare. The reason I recommend this is because ADD medications often require *titration*, or adjustments, so that they will continue to work well for the patient over time with little or no side effects. And 10 or 15 minutes is just not enough time to discuss your medication and determine whether or not it is the correct dose, or even the correct medicine!

Once you have a psychiatrist whom you like, respect, and trust, and your medication is working well for you, your psychiatrist may be willing to work with you to keep the expenses down. For example, they may see you for shorter visits most of the year, and extended visits every few months. Or, they may feel comfortable letting your general practitioner prescribe your refills, and allow you to see them every couple of months.

Bonus Tip: If your budget is a concern when finding a good psychiatrist for your ADD medication, then take the time to take a few extra steps:

Find out if your insurance company will reimburse you for all or part of your out-of-pocket expenses for a visit to a psychiatrist who doesn't take insurance.

Talk to your psychiatrist about your situation. They may be able to work with your budget, or refer you to someone whom they trust, but charges less.

Cut down on luxuries, like restaurant dinners or new clothes, in order to afford top-notch healthcare by a psychiatrist you like, respect, and trust.

If you'd like to search online for a psychiatrist or other health care professional who has experience treating adults with ADD, then visit the Odd One Out Reader's Resources webpage at **www.odd-one-out.net/resources.html** for a list of online directories.

5. Don't Be Afraid to Say "Screw 'em!"

When you begin slowing down, taking care of yourself, and managing your stress, you can fully expect some people in your life to become combative. You can expect that they will push back against your new boundaries and even criticize your efforts to take care of yourself first. Screw 'em.

People who don't take care of themselves

will feel threatened by you when you begin putting yourself first. They won't understand why they feel threatened and they may not even be aware of it. But you can expect to feel a squeeze. Don't take it personally and, whatever you do, don't feel guilty! Take a good look at the people giving you a hassle. I can guarantee they aren't the maverick types! I'll bet that they spend a lot of energy following the rules and aren't very happy in their own lives. Which is unfortunate, but it's not your problem. All you can do is take care of you. Do what you know is right for you.

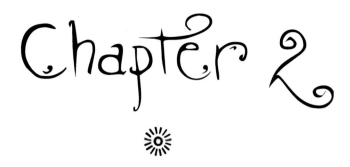

Work With Your ADD, Not Against It

OTHER PEOPLE'S RULES DON'T WORK

Adults with ADD spend a lot of time trying to fit in by doing things the way they *think* other people do them. We try to play by other people's rules, and it often doesn't work.

In order to embrace your maverick nature and use it to your advantage, you have to stop being concerned about whether or not you do things the way everyone else does. What everyone else does is irrelevant. What works for *you* is what matters.

The trouble with following other people's rules is that other people don't have ADD! They aren't hardwired the way you are. So playing the game of life according to someone else's rules will almost always have you working *against* your ADD, when it's much more efficient, and much less stressful, to work with it.

In this chapter, we're going to talk about building awareness of your own ADD challenges, and calling on your maverick nature to work with your natural tendencies.

DON'T TRUST YOUR JUDGMENT

You've probably spent a lifetime paying attention to your differences and kicking yourself for them. In our society, we're often taught that *different* equals *bad*. Your parents may have called you lazy because you had no interest in cleaning your room. Your teachers may have told you that you didn't apply yourself because you daydreamed in class. And your friends may have commented that you never paid attention to the rules of the game. These behaviors in and of themselves aren't *bad*, just *different* than those of most other kids.

These early experiences become internalized, whether or not you're aware of them. And in adulthood it gets worse, because *you* do most of the comparisons. Suddenly you're noticing all the ways in which you don't measure up. You have the messiest desk in the whole office. You forget to go to the grocery store and have no food in the fridge. You show up late to the party because you can't find your keys. You're the odd one out. And the whole time you keep telling yourself, *No one else seems to have these problems. What's wrong with me?*

There is nothing wrong with scattering your

desk with papers, forgetting to run an errand, or misplacing an object. Sure, all these things can be annoying, but there is nothing inherently *bad* about any of them. So why do you beat yourself up about it? **As long as you continue to judge yourself for your differences, you're working against your ADD.** Keep this in mind as you begin building your awareness around your particular ADD-related traits. Don't get down on yourself simply because you do things differently from other people. Build your awareness objectively and *without judgment.*

Sharon's Story

As far back as she could remember, Sharon was critical of herself. She was told that she was too slow and didn't try hard enough in school. She believed it. She didn't do very well in school, and she often felt stupid.

As an adult, Sharon was constantly frustrated with herself. She was always pressed for time and everything felt like a hassle. She felt guilty when she misplaced something or let piles build up on her desk.

In her late 40s, and with a husband and 2 kids, Sharon went back to school. This time around, she did well! But she didn't give herself credit for it because she felt that it took her too long to obtain her degree.

A decade later, Sharon was diagnosed with ADD, and so was her son. She wanted to learn everything she could about ADD and how to manage it, and she became one of my early coaching clients.

Everything changed for Sharon when she got to know her own ADD. She was able to accept her forgetfulness and her need to be a bit disorganized because there was a reason for it. She wasn't being lazy or not trying hard enough. Her brain just worked differently, and even though she might be able to create systems and improve situations, she had no control over how her brain was wired. For the first time in her life, she understood that her challenges weren't her fault.

Sharon still gets frustrated over things, but she can now stand up for herself and tell people, "This is the best I can do, and if it's not good enough for you, too bad."

She understands which challenges are related to ADD, and she refuses to fall apart over them. She lets go of frustrations easier. She feels comfortable asking for help in the areas where she's not strong. She no longer gets in her own way.

Inspired by the positive changes she made in herself, Sharon decided to become an ADD Coach, too. She now works with me in the ADD Management Group and coaches clients on the skills that she learned and applied for herself.

Today, Sharon's motto is "don't let what you can't do get in the way of what you can." She believes it, and she lives it.

Have you ever been told that you're your own

worst enemy? It's a common statement made to adults with ADD by the people who love them.

One of the biggest mistakes that adults with ADD make is that they hold themselves to unrealistic expectations. When your expectations of yourself are unrealistic, you simply can't win. As a result, your self-esteem will always be in the gutter.

You are who you are. You, like all people, have both weaknesses and strengths. You have challenges, problems, and "issues." You also have talents, strengths, skills, and passions. Together, these traits combine to make you the person you are. Mavericks understand that who you are is not good or bad, it just is.

And just as it's necessary to be aware of your strengths (which we'll talk about in the next chapter), it's necessary to be aware of your challenges. This awareness serves a very important purpose: it acts as a guide for you as you use your maverick nature to make your own rules.

This means that you play your own game based on what works for you, *not* what works for other people. The only way to achieve this is to be objective and neutral about your shortcomings. Challenges are neither good nor bad. They are neutral. Judging them only gives them power and lowers your self-esteem.

Of course ADDers struggle with challenges. But with time, experimentation, and a positive attitude, you can take the good stuff, and use it to overcome the not-so-good stuff. **When**

you begin to look at what's right with you, and what you are capable of under the right circumstances, you open up a world of possibilities. Knowing yourself well, and thus knowing your ADD well, means looking at a complete picture of yourself and embracing it all.

Mavericks know who they are and what they want, and don't judge themselves for any of it!

WHAT IS AND ISN'T ADD?

This is a great question, considering that many experts disagree on what ADD is, who it affects, and the symptoms it presents.

The current *Diagnostic and Statistical Manual* (DSM-IV) that doctors use to diagnose "mental disorders" lists 3 types of ADD: predominantly inattentive, predominantly hyperactive-impulsive, and combined type. I've read books and seen presentations by doctors and researchers who believe that each type of ADD is its own particular "disorder." I've also seen experts who think that all 3 types are one and the same. Sometimes I think the only thing we know for sure about ADD is that all the experts disagree about it!

Through all the disagreements, however, it is evident that adults with ADD do share similar challenges. The most commonly associated challenges are hyperactivity, inattention, and impulsivity. But there are some lesser-known

WORK WITH YOUR ADD, NOT AGAINST IT

challenges that adults with ADD experience, many of them dealing with what we call "executive functioning."

Executive functioning is the term used to describe the brain's system of managing the tasks of day-to-day life. Planning, organization, and time management are all executive functions.

Some of the lesser-known challenges of adult ADD oftentimes have the biggest impact on ADDers. In large part, this is simply because no one talks about these challenges. If you find that you are emotionally reactive when frustrated, but your friends and family are not, you may be tempted to think that there is something wrong with you.

Because emotional reactivity is not necessarily a desirable behavior and may be something that you'd like to work on improving, it can be hard to accept this tendency without judgment or bad feelings. But this is actually a common trait among adults with ADD. Simply knowing this—that you are not alone in your struggles to manage your emotions—can take a huge amount of pressure off and allow you to objectively build your awareness.

So let's take a look at some common ADD challenges and how they might affect you. The goal of this section is to help you build personal awareness, so as you read through the next few pages, try to determine the challenges that you face and perhaps make some notes about them.

HYPERACTIVITY

Adults with ADD often experience hyperactivity. Hyperactivity can take many forms. Adults who are physically hyperactive may experience:

- A desire to be constantly going and doing
- A tendency to fidget and an inability to sit still
- Extreme boredom when forced to wait for something or when being in one place for too long

Hyperactivity can also be mental. Although many adults with ADD don't experience physical hyperactivity, most do experience mental hyperactivity, such as:

- A racing mind that won't calm down or shut off, even when the body is tired or sedentary
- Nagging thoughts about what you should or shouldn't do
- Continually thinking up and planning ideas and next steps, sometimes without intention or outside prompting

Some adults with ADD "idle" higher than others and are capable of getting more done in a day than most people, which is a nice benefit! And mavericks can use hyperactivity to their advantage. It can provide fuel to get important things done and to think up elaborate or creative plans.

But the ADD maverick needs to be careful, because hyperactivity can have some pretty negative effects. For one, it wears you down. When your body and/or mind is constantly running and doing, it's easy to become tired and overwhelmed.

And the racing brain that we experience in mental hyperactivity often lends itself to negative and judgmental thoughts. It's not uncommon for the hyperactive brain to spend a large chunk of time ruminating over mistakes and problems. Maverick ADDers need to have a keen awareness of their hyperactive minds, and take steps to slow them down when they turn to nagging, negative thoughts, or overwhelm.

INATTENTION

Adults with ADD experience a paradox when it comes to paying attention. The term "Attention Deficit Disorder" is actually quite misleading when you consider that we don't really have a deficit of attention. Rather, we have *attention inconsistencies*. **Probably the greatest ADD paradox is the fact that we can lose focus in times of boredom, and focus intensely during times of interest.** Typical experiences include:

- An inability to concentrate, even when you're really trying to

- Being easily distracted, annoyed, or frustrated
- An inability to smoothly shift focus when appropriate
- Becoming easily bored
- Daydreaming or "zoning out"
- Having to reread information several times before taking it in and understanding it
- Focusing so intently that you lose track of time or forget important things
- Becoming temporarily obsessed with information or subjects of interest
- Improved focus under pressure or deadlines

Attention and focus problems are particularly challenging for adults at work and in the classroom. We're often asked to perform tasks or attend to projects that we have little interest in, and it can be hard to control your mind and keep it focused when you're bored.

Additionally, many adults with ADD find that they zone out during meetings or important conversations without even realizing it! This can be both troublesome and embarrassing. Your maverick nature may have you wanting to say "Screw this!" and moving onto better things, but sometimes we have no choice and have to play by someone else's rules. It's not nice to tell off your great Aunt Edna no matter how boring she is, and informing the boss that you'd rather play solitaire than attend another meeting could get you fired.

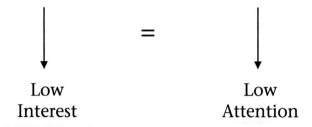

The good news is that there is a powerful paradox at work when it comes to attention. While we can become easily bored and distracted when uninterested, we can *hyper-focus* when we are interested.

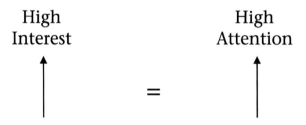

As a maverick who likes to make your own rules, this is a trait that can prove to be highly beneficial. When an ADDer becomes hyper-focused on something important, look out! Chances are you will perform very well and achieve success—if you can keep from burning out.

And let's not forget that the spacey, daydreaming element of adult ADD is actually quite creative. When you daydream, you are paying attention—you're just not paying attention to what is happening around you in that moment. Instead, you're very much alive and focused on the interesting world inside your head! If the rest of the world could see the things you dream up, they'd be impressed.

If you really want to nurture the maverick inside you, let those daydreams loose on the world! Try turning them into a form of creative or artistic expression.

IMPULSIVITY

Impulsivity in adults with ADD can take many forms. Some common examples are:

- Talking without thinking your words through, leading to embarrassment or regret
- Making snap decisions that may not be in your best interest
- Over-committing your time and energy in an effort to please
- Difficulty avoiding damaging behaviors, like impulsive shopping, drinking, gambling, and other potentially addictive actions
- Engaging in potentially dangerous thrill-seeking behavior

Impulsivity can be highly damaging when you speak before thinking. You can end up offending people, giving away too much information, and making promises that you can't easily keep. Mavericks need to remember that self-care comes first. This sometimes means holding your tongue when you really want to spill your guts.

Impulsivity can also be a positive trait. For example, many adults with ADD are known among their friends and family as being fun and spontaneous. New ideas are plentiful, and are often backed up with intense energy.

Mavericks have to be careful to balance impulsivity with a little foresight. It can be very easy to jump on a new idea, only to find that it doesn't interest you in the long run. Having a plan to follow through can be helpful.

Or, you can just embrace your impulsive nature and accept that you will probably always be jumping from one interest to the next. If this sounds like you, then it's wise not to spend a lot of money on new hobbies if there is a chance you will shortly drop them in favor of a new interest.

TAKING ACTION

Moving from thought to action can be quite difficult for ADDers. Some common challenges in this area include:

- Prolonged and frequent periods of procrastination
- Trouble activating or getting started during the day
- Trouble activating or getting started on individual tasks
- Difficulty prioritizing tasks
- An inability to organize physical spaces and/or mental thoughts
- Trouble making and trusting decisions, both large and small

- An inability to create and stick to effective structure
- Difficulty attending to details
- Boredom with the minutia of day-to-day life

While this area of challenge is not often talked about, it's the one that is the most damaging for many adults with ADD. As children, the thought-to-action process is often taken care of for us: your parents told you when to get up, when to go to bed, when to eat, when to clean your room, and when to do your homework. Your teachers instructed you what to work on in school, and what to work on at home. Your sports coach or dance teacher told you what to practice.

As an adult, you're on your own. For the most part, no one tells you when to get out of bed in the morning or forces you to turn off the TV and go to bed at night. No one reminds you that it's lunch time. The boss doesn't prioritize your to-do list, and doesn't sit with you while you complete your work.

As a result, adults with ADD commonly go through the day feeling overwhelmed by all that has to be done, and not knowing when or how to do it all. As seen in the last chapter, this overwhelm tends to shut down the ADD brain, which in turn makes prioritizing, organizing, decision making, and taking action in general more difficult.

So without an effectively prioritized to-do list, the work builds up, which may lead to overwhelm and procrastination. And sometimes the more you put off that work, the harder it seems to get started. Without effective organization systems, confusion builds and spaces become even more disorganized. Similarly, the longer a decision is put off and pondered over, the bigger it seems and the harder it becomes to make a decision.

In all these situations, the brain is on high speed, thinking about all that needs to be done or put into action. **The more thinking you do, the harder action becomes.** Mavericks need to step back sometimes and allow room to put everything in perspective. We'll discuss this in detail in Chapter 4.

On a positive note, many ADDers believe that this disorganization of space and mind may actually promote creativity. And mavericks are often creative, big-picture thinkers, which can be an asset in many areas of life.

MEMORY

It's widely accepted that ADD doesn't affect long-term memory, but it does affect short-term, or working, memory. Some examples include:

- Forgetting where you put your keys, cell phone, wallet, and other objects
- Frequently losing things and unexpectedly finding things
- Struggling to remember names, faces, or other "details"
- Walking into a room and realizing that you

have no idea what you went in there for
- Feeling overwhelmed by too much information, too many distractions, or too much
stimuli

These working memory problems are extremely
frustrating and annoying. Slowing down certainly
helps improve these problems. If you're constantly
in chaos mode, then of course there will be many
little details that slip from your memory.

Custom-created systems can be helpful. For
example, if you're constantly losing your keys,
create a spot for them and train yourself to always
put them there.

Mavericks can learn to accept that their working memory won't be as sharp as other people's
sometimes, and deal with it. In fact, these working memory problems often result in some good
"ADD moments." And if you can't laugh at yourself, then you're really in trouble!

Here are some of the better "ADD moments" that
have been told to me by clients and colleagues:

- Misplacing a cell phone in the vegetable
crisper
- Throwing the car keys in the garbage and
throwing the garbage on the counter
- Showing up to a doctor's appointment one
day early
- Showing up to a dentist's appointment one
month late
- Spending an entire evening searching for

lost keys that were on the key rack the whole time
- Creating a detailed to-do list, and losing it an hour later
- Fighting with a cashier about getting the wrong change for a $20 bill, only to discover that a $10 bill was used to pay
- Being chased by a waiter for forgetting to pay the bill before leaving the restaurant
- Missing the "handicapped parking space" sign and getting a ticket for being parked illegally (that one's mine)

ADD moments are usually harmless and, while they can be stressful, they can often provide a good laugh.

ALERTNESS

One of the lesser-known challenges of adult ADD is an inconsistency in alertness and energy levels. Many adults with ADD experience:

- Difficulty falling asleep at night
- Trouble waking up or getting out of bed in the morning
- A need to "ease into" the day
- Feeling sleepy and groggy when you need to be awake and alert
- Feeling awake and alert when you need to be winding down and relaxing

- Difficulty following through on projects because energy levels start out high but quickly decrease
- Trouble absorbing or understanding information because of low energy

These issues with alertness and energy regulation might not be a big deal if the rest of the world didn't operate on a strict schedule. But most ADDers are forced to abandon their natural biorhythms in order to operate in a world that is largely 9-to-5. And energy regulation can be extremely troublesome at work or school when you're forced to conform to other people's timelines and energy levels.

Although these inconsistencies in alertness and energy regulation can prove quite troublesome, many ADDers find that if they are able to tune into and honor their own biorhythms, they do quite well. In fact, lots of artistic ADDers report that an "up all night, sleep all day" schedule solidly supports their creative process.

Mavericks need to work with their own biorhythms as much as possible. That means taking advantage of the times in which your brain is most alert, and not trying to squeeze too much out of yourself during the times when you're naturally less energetic. Again, we'll discuss this further in Chapter 4.

EMOTIONAL SENSITIVITY AND REACTIVITY

This is a subject that really needs to be discussed. You don't hear about it often, yet it is one of the great challenges of adult ADD. It wreaks havoc in the lives of many ADDers, and so many don't even know that their emotional reactivity is linked to their ADD!

Adults with ADD tend to be highly sensitive and emotional. This becomes a problem when you're overwhelmed and frustrated, because it is more difficult to control your thoughts, feelings, and emotions when your brain feels like it's operating at full capacity. It's not at all uncommon for adults with ADD to experience:

- A tendency to become very easily frustrated or overwhelmed
- Very strong emotions that seem to be uncontrollable
- A state of extreme agitation in which little things prove to be unbearably annoying
- Taking out anger, sadness, disappointment, and other negative emotions on those closest to you, and for "no good reason"
- Being extremely upset by criticism or negative feedback
- Extreme self-judgment because of the tendency to become easily frustrated and overly emotional

The more stressed out and frustrated you are,

the more likely you are to experience extreme emotional states. The emotions themselves are never bad; emotions are part of being human and allowing yourself to experience your emotions fully is actually very healthy. The problems mainly come into play when 1) other people become involved and 2) you judge yourself so severely and harshly for your emotions that you label yourself a "bad person."

Getting a piece of negative feedback at work can be further complicated if you instantly react with uncontrollable sobbing. Becoming frustrated when trying to fix your broken stereo can be further complicated when you snap at your kids for interrupting you. And judging yourself for what seem to be automatic and unnecessary emotional reactions can just make you more overwhelmed and stressed out, not to mention sad.

There is, however, an upside to this trait. Emotionally sensitive ADDers have a strong sense of empathy and compassion. We tend to be do-gooders who genuinely care about people. We have the ability to see multiple points of view, and to imagine how we would feel in another's place. These are strong character traits that continually make the world a better place.

Mavericks allow themselves to feel their emotions fully and without judgment. They strive to express these emotions in a healthy way, and use their emotional nature to make sincere connections with other people.

Mavericks honor who they are without trying to be someone else. Working *with* your ADD means that you know who you are, and you accept who you are. You may identify areas of your life in which you want to improve, but for the most part you commit to working with your individual characteristics and qualities—whether they are "challenges" or "advantages."

The science behind ADD is fascinating. If you're interested in reading more about the ADD brain and how adult ADD may affect you, visit the Odd One Out Reader's Resources webpage at **www.odd-one-out.net/resources.html.**

PAY ATTENTION!

It's absolutely necessary to embrace your differences when you need to pay attention and take in information. As an adult with ADD, you have no doubt noticed that when most people need to chill out and pay attention, they seem to be able to do so with little trouble, while you have great difficulty. Meetings, classrooms, and even boring conversations can be awful experiences for ADDers!

Jimmy's Story

As a kid, Jimmy was hyperactive. He was a jokester in school, and didn't like to stay still. In high school, Jimmy developed an annoying habit that drove his family crazy: he constantly bounced a tennis ball.

It didn't matter if he was doing his homework,

talking to his parents, or watching TV. He always had a ball in one hand and he would bounce it on the most convenient surface—the floor, a wall, a table.

His mother didn't approve of bouncing balls in the house, but more than anything, the noise was incredibly annoying and distracting to the rest of his family!

But Jimmy was barely aware of what he was doing. All he knew was that he couldn't focus without that ball. He struggled in class without his ball, and he would get in trouble for fidgeting too much.

It all made sense once Jimmy got to college. He was studying to be a teacher and learned all about the different modalities that people engaged during the learning process. He realized through his coursework that he had ADD, and that sometimes, hyperactive kids with ADD need to move around to pay attention. Suddenly, the tennis ball made sense!

Armed with this new knowledge, Jimmy found other ways to pay attention—ways that didn't disturb the people around him. His job as a teacher is great because it allows him to interact and engage with his students all day. And when he does have to sit still in meetings, he uses small fidget toys to keep occupied. He's found a way to work with his ADD and pay attention when he needs to.

You'll no doubt have the hardest time paying attention when you try to force yourself to do it.

That simply doesn't work for ADDers. Boredom sets in and your mind wanders when you're not even noticing!

It's often necessary to activate the part of your brain that allows you to buck up and pay attention. It may not be what other people do, but mavericks do what works! Some ADDers find that when trying to pay attention, they need to do one or more of the following:

1. Get Physical
Fidgeting, doodling, standing, stretching, eating, drinking, swiveling in your chair, and other types of movement help many ADDers pay attention.

One thing to consider here is that if you need to move in order to focus and pay attention, you can easily become a distraction or an annoyance to those around you. Try to find a form of movement that helps you stay focused without interrupting others' concentration.

2. Get Visual
Some ADDers find that visual stimulation allows them to pay better attention. This may mean focusing on visual cues, like colors or written words.

I once had a client who was so bored in her college classes that she would nearly fall asleep. When she started experimenting with methods for paying better attention, she began bringing colorful pictures and drawings into her classes. She found that simply being able to stare at the colors while listening activated her brain enough for her to pay attention without becoming bored.

3. Get Audio

There are some ADDers out there who find that intense listening is what allows them to focus on and absorb information. For these ADDers, it can be necessary to block out all distractions and focus on what a person is saying.

In this case, audio recordings of meetings, classes, and other important information can prove to be extremely valuable.

Conversely, some auditory ADDers find that *adding music* or other background noise can help improve concentration!

I encourage you to experiment with these different strategies so that you get to know which work best for you in different situations. Mavericks understand that they don't always pay attention in the same way others do. They aren't concerned with being different or looking silly.

If you encounter objections—from your boss, teacher, or anyone else—simply explain yourself. There is nothing wrong with explaining that you find it easier to pay close attention when you stand up during a meeting. As long as you're not bothering anyone else, there shouldn't be any objections from the powers that be.

EXPRESS YOURSELF

Another important element of working with your ADD is to understand the best and easiest ways for you to *unload* information. I call this "clearing the mental clutter."

Adults with ADD are subjected to more stimuli and distractions than the average person, and therefore finding a way to stop paying attention can be just as important as learning how to pay attention in the first place! Unloading excess information and negative thoughts goes a long way towards managing stress and overwhelm. In fact, I recommend that you regularly take time to process and release all the thoughts that are hanging around in your head. This is especially true during times of stress and overwhelm!

And in the same way that ADDers pay attention differently than most, we may also need to unload differently, too. Here are some different ways that you can work through thoughts and feelings that seem hard to let go of:

1. Move It
Release your stress and frustration with movement. Use a vigorous workout to relieve your stress, or take a leisurely stroll to clear your head.

2. Write It
I highly recommend journaling for ADD management. It's a great way to process your thoughts, feelings, and frustrations.

Additionally, making lists, creating mind maps or brainstorms, writing poetry, and other forms of putting pen to paper can provide great relief for a cluttered mind.

3. Speak It
You can also try verbally processing your thoughts. When something is sitting heavy on your mind, talk to a friend, family member, therapist, coach, or anyone else who will listen.

You can even talk to your pets or speak into a voice recorder! If you get relief from verbal processing, it doesn't matter what you say or who you say it to. The benefit is derived from actually *talking out* your thoughts and feelings.

COMMUNICATING YOUR DIFFERENCES TO OTHERS

The key to working with your ADD is really just allowing yourself to be who you are—challenges, quirks, and all. And if you run into resistance from a boss, spouse, family member, or anyone else, don't be afraid to use this phrase: *I work best when* ____.

If you get feedback or criticism from people who don't understand why you are the way you are or why you do certain things the way you do them, don't backtrack.

Don't apologize, don't justify, and don't try to change simply because someone else doesn't understand you. Just explain that you work best when _____.

So if your spouse wants to know how you can read with the TV on, just explain, "I actually read better when I have some background noise."

If your boss complains that your doodling in meetings means that you're not paying attention, simply explain, "I pay attention best when I can fidget."

Mavericks know that when you embrace yourself as the *total package,* your confidence will radiate and others will accept you, too.

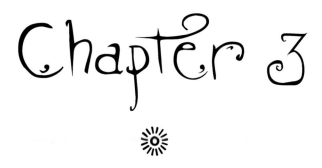

Chapter 3

ADDjust Your Attitude

YOUR BAD ATTITUDE GETS YOU NOWHERE

Trying to follow other people's rules, especially when those rules aren't a good fit for you, will quickly diminish your self-esteem. How can you feel good about yourself when you're trying to squeeze into a narrow mold that was made for someone else? *Mavericks break the mold!*

Being a happy and successful adult with ADD requires you to do 2 things: focus on your strengths, and maintain a positive attitude.

HOW DO WE BECOME SO NEGATIVE?

I usually begin my conversations with new clients by saying, "Tell me about yourself and why you're looking for coaching." Most people answer with a long list of their ADD challenges. Very few people answer that they are looking to discover, enhance, or utilize their strengths. This is a big part of the reason why many adults with ADD need help in the first place.

Danielle's Story

Danielle survived an abusive household and a parent with severe mental illness. She went back to school and got an advanced degree as an adult. She overcame drug and alcohol addiction and is now 17 years sober. She's been happily partnered for 16 years. She has strong friendships. She's a gifted social worker. She is open minded, energetic, enthusiastic, driven, kind hearted, and funny. **She's clearly one of the most resilient people you'll ever meet.** *But when I first started working with Danielle, she couldn't see any of that.*

Instead, she saw a person who had nothing to offer the world. She focused heavily on the poor choices she made in her youth. She echoed the negative feedback she had received as a kid—that she was disorganized, lazy, stupid, scattered, and going nowhere.

Danielle always firmly believed in her mission

as a social worker: to help people understand their strengths and achieve their highest level of performance. Yet she didn't think the same standards applied to her.

Despite enduring tremendous hardships and obstacles in her life, Danielle always maintained a little light of hope. She was open minded, and willing to give the coaching process a chance. We worked intensively on building her self-esteem, and it wasn't easy for her.

We started small. Each week, she would send me an email telling me what she did right that week. It was hard for her to focus on her strengths and what was going well, but she committed to it. Some weeks I'd get an email that said nothing more than "My only accomplishment this week is actually sitting down to send this email." It was something.

Slowly but surely, she started to notice her accomplishments. Getting a Master's Degree with honors was wonderful. But the little things were important, too. She started paying attention to the compliments that she would receive at work. She became proud of herself when she cleaned up her office, rather than getting down on herself for messing it up in the first place. And once she started focusing on the good stuff, the good stuff in her life multiplied. For the first time, she was able to see just how resilient she was. She was able to turn off all those old tapes that played in her head, telling her what a bad person she was. She began to appreciate her own strengths and good qualities.

*She has confidence now, and because she isn't
so critical of herself anymore, she's actually enjoying her life. Her reviews at work have never been
better. She now accepts compliments instead of
fighting them. And she is exploring her creative
talents in ways that she never before allowed herself to. She is a happier, lighter person.*

 *Danielle now has a mission in life. She's fo-
cused on using her people skills to change the face
of her particular branch of social work. She has
a plan, and she thinks that she can make a real
difference in the world.*

 I know she can.

So many ADDers spend too much of their time
focusing on what they think they do wrong.
This is understandable, as most of us have spent
a lifetime learning how to deal with our ADD
challenges and differences. If, as a child (and as
an adult), you received a lot of negative feedback about being "lazy," "slow," "disorganized,"
"spacey," or similar, then you have probably internalized this feedback and think these things
about yourself.

 Similarly, if you were called out for being different, you probably internalized this as being bad.
Unfortunately, in our culture, different equals
bad. It's no fun being the odd one out when
you're a kid.

 It's easy to believe these messages, especially
when you're young. They often become ingrained
and until they are dealt with properly, tapes of

these old messages will play over and over again in times of stress and self-doubt.

Sometimes the self-criticism we develop really is based in reality because, as humans, we do have weaknesses, challenges, issues and problems. No one is perfect, and no one can be good at everything...and that's a good thing!

In the United States and many other cultures, the prevailing thought is that weaknesses need to be turned into strengths. When an area of weakness or challenge is identified, you're supposed to "fix it" by willpower and self-control. So if you're not very organized, you're supposed to become a neat freak. If you tend to run late, you're supposed to learn how to be early.

But it's all just bullshit.

Organized and early are considered "good" qualities. Being disorganized and late has no value. But what if this prevailing "wisdom" is all wrong? What if there is a place for all of these undesirable qualities that does, in fact, make them desirable?

In order to answer this question, let's first take a look at some common ADD strengths. While everyone is different, there is a set of positive characteristics that I frequently observe in adults with ADD.

1. Creativity

I've never met an ADDer who wasn't creative in one way or another. Being creative does not necessarily mean being artistic, although that very well may be the case. There are tons of ADDers who are writers, painters, performers, photographers, and so on.

Other ADDers are problem solvers. They enjoy taking a problem and finding unconventional or unobvious ways to solve it.

Some are innovative and strategic thinkers. They are really good at coming up with new ideas and planning out how to implement them. There are a lot of ADDers out there who are entrepreneurs and inventors and tech wizards—the ultimate mavericks who push the limits, break the rules, and move society forward.

2. Compassion

ADDers are people-people. We tend to have extremely high levels of empathy and compassion. (In fact, this can sometimes hurt an adult with ADD who gets caught up in feeling another's pain *too* deeply.)

The ADDers I know generally "do the right thing," like return found wallets or help an older stranger climb some stairs. They are usually the go-to person among friends and family when someone has a problem and needs a friend or a sympathetic ear.

This quality also makes many ADDers great sales people because we are usually more motivated by helping a person than by making a sale just for the sake of it.

And lots of other adults with ADD can be found in helping professions, like healthcare and social work.

3. Drive

When an ADDer sets their mind on an important goal, look out! This drive to succeed may not always be evident because it often requires an intense desire or passion to come to the forefront, but when called up, that drive will take a person far.

4. Resiliency

Everyone experiences tragedy, hardship, and disappointments. It's a part of life. And adults with ADD arguably have more difficulties than others due to our common challenges. But we also have great strength and resiliency.

ADDers often feel pain and disappointment, but tend to have an amazing capacity to jump back into the game and move forward. The next time you think back on mistakes you made or things you're not proud of, also think about what it took for you to pick up and move past the problems!

Of course, adults with ADD have many more strengths and talents, but these are the 4 that I truly believe we *all* have in common. It's a short list, but a powerful one that is full of highly desirable qualities.

So now, let me ask you, would you rather be creative, compassionate, driven, resilient, disorganized, and late...

Or would you rather be organized, early, unimaginative, unfeeling, lazy, and weak?

Give me the former any day.

If you're not convinced, then try an example that makes more sense to you. Quickly determine 3 things that you struggle with. Then ask yourself, would you rather conquer those 3 challenges in exchange for giving up being creative, compassionate, driven, and resilient? Would you rather trade in your strengths for mastery of your weaknesses? I certainly wouldn't.

The point is that no one is perfect. We all have strengths and we all have weaknesses. **And when you look at yourself as a whole picture, instead of isolating and focusing on your weaknesses, suddenly those weaknesses don't have quite so much power.**

Consider this: most organized people are not very creative. Organized people tend to be extremely detail-oriented and creative people tend to be more big-picture thinkers. It's pretty hard to be good at both these things. And while you're wishing you were organized, tons of organized people are wishing they were creative.

The world goes 'round because different people fill different roles. If everyone were organized, the world would be pretty boring. There would be a lack of art and innovation. And if everyone were creative, nothing would ever get done! So if you're a creative person, stop kicking yourself for being disorganized. The world needs *both* organized people *and* creative people.

IT DOESN'T NEED TO BE FIXED

Carrie's Story

Sometimes your life has to fall apart in order for you to build it back up the way you want it to be. This is what happened to Carrie.

Her relationship was in trouble. She had an affair that ended badly for all involved, and caused a lot of emotional turmoil. And the weight of it all was causing Carrie to suffer at work. She was overwhelmed and disorganized.

As a therapist, she was there for her clients. But she had no motivation to return phone calls, schedule appointments, or complete necessary paperwork. She wasn't even getting her time sheets completed in time to be paid! She felt completely depleted. And she knew that the only way to make things better was to get out of her head and take action.

In coaching, Carrie felt validated. She knew that she wasn't lazy or a bad person, but she needed to hear it. She needed to be reminded that the problems she was having at work were related to her ADD. And that, of course, the more stressed she was, the worse her challenges became.

Carrie assessed herself and her life with a newfound clarity. She had to accept who she was and where she was at before she could make changes. She knew there was a way to harness her positive traits while taking her challenges into account. She began looking at her career in the framework of her ADD, and decided that her job in a big therapy partnership didn't suit her well. She felt like a talented and creative person, and her clients loved her. But she was tired of being judged for the little things she had trouble with, like running a few minutes late here and there, or needing a little extra time for paperwork.

Through this acceptance of herself, she felt motivated and empowered to explore her gifts and her quirkiness. She found a new job that was perfect for her. In addition to working with clients, she was supervising a staff and found that the role suited her well. She was using her creative strengths, and she realized that she's a much better leader than follower. Her new job was also more structured and, because she was expected to maintain a minimum number of office hours, the paperwork no longer seemed like a chore.

Little by little, the other aspects of Carrie's life also fell into place. It became clear that her relationship was not working, and she ended it. It felt like a good decision. She also began exploring her creative talents outside of work, getting back to her passion for writing music, and even starting a small crafts business.

Yes, Carrie had a very difficult time for a while. But she allowed herself to feel the pain, and to put all the pieces back in just the way she wanted them. She did so not by trying to fix what was wrong, but by focusing on what was right.

I'm not suggesting that there isn't room for improvement when it comes to our weaknesses and challenges. Certainly, becoming more organized is a worthwhile goal. Getting to appointments on time is a worthwhile goal.

A serious problem presents itself, however, when you try to "fix" a weakness. Here's why: no one ever became successful by focusing on eliminating their challenges. **People become successful when they focus on, and build upon, the things they're already good at.**

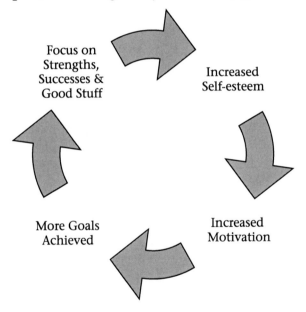

Think about it: if you waste all your time trying to become ultra organized, perfectly manage your time, and squeeze your body into a mold that it doesn't fit, you don't get very far. Most of the time, you can perhaps sharpen those weaknesses to the point where they become neutral and you are neither good nor bad at them.

But in the time that it takes to become neutral in your weak areas, you could instead focus on becoming *really sharp* at the things you're already good at. You can enhance your strengths and hone your talents.

A musician doesn't sell records by learning how to get to an appointment on time; they sell records by becoming a really good musician!

Certainly, putting a little effort towards being on time will help in their career, but it's not going to get them the big break.

A marketer doesn't get promoted by being the person in the office with the best filing system; they get promoted by being a good marketer!

Having an organized office may impress the boss and win some brownie points, but ultimately, the boss cares about the results that are produced.

An artist doesn't get their work displayed in a gallery because they go to bed early every night; they get their work displayed by being a good artist!

Getting a good night's sleep is definitely important and will help anyone be on top of their game, but early to bed and early to rise doesn't make an artist.

You get the point. Improving on weaknesses is great, but don't focus on weaknesses. Mavericks focus on their strengths.

BUT I DON'T EVEN KNOW WHAT I'M GOOD AT

Unfortunately, I hear this from a lot of ADDers. If you really don't know what you're good at, then I suggest 3 things:

1. Ask the people you trust. You'll be pleasantly surprised when you see that the people closest to you generally agree on what you're good at.
2. Pay attention to the compliments people give you. Say thank you and take the positive feedback.
3. Identify your interests and the things you're passionate about. Somewhere in these, you'll find what you're good at.

DON'T BE A BMW

"BMW" is short for someone who bitches, moans, and whines. BMWs never get anywhere in life. They're too busy complaining and finding problems with *everything*. They don't take responsibility for their actions and choices, and instead blame others for their mistakes. They're a drag. They suck the energy right out of you, and leave you feeling pretty crappy about the world, and yourself! You know the type. *Or maybe you are one?*

I can understand how people with ADD can become BMWs. You spent a lifetime feeling different and being the odd one out. You've probably had your share of criticism like "you're lazy," "you don't try hard enough," "you make careless mistakes," "you could do so much better if you only *applied* yourself," and much worse. And these experiences may have caused you to develop some bitter, cynical tendencies. But staying bitter and cynical is your choice. So is moving beyond it.

It didn't take long for me to notice BMWs in my coaching clients. They are the most difficult people to work with because they don't trust you, they don't trust the process, and they don't trust themselves. In group situations, they ruin the experience for others by being negative, pessimistic, and closed-minded. BMWs are downers! And BMWs have to get over their bitching, moaning, and whining if they want to learn how to manage their ADD and embrace the maverick within.

Are You a BMW?

If you answer "yes" to 2 or more of the following questions, then you very well may be a BMW!

- Do you often see the bad in situations before you see the good?
- Do you constantly find fault with the people around you?
- Has anyone ever told you that you complain too much?
- Do you think you're right all the time?

If you think that you might be a BMW, don't fret.

I used to be one, too. In fact, I still catch myself re-
verting back to old tendencies sometimes, and have
to remind myself that my attitude needs adjusting!
**BMWs are really just negative thinkers
without the tools, and sometimes the will-
ingness, to change their thinking patterns.**
If you're willing to become a more positive and
happy person, then you can begin immediately.
If you think that "positive thinking" is a bunch
of New Age crap, then I encourage you to remain
open minded as you read the following pages because, clearly, *you are a negative thinker*!

FORMS OF NEGATIVE THINKING

If you pay attention to your own negative thinking patterns, you'll find that 99% of your negative
thoughts are about one of 2 things:

1. Worrying in the form of "What am I going
   to do if (insert any undesirable circumstance)
   happens?"
2. "What will/do (insert name of any person or
   group of people) think of me?"

I understand the first example all too well, partly
because I come from a long line of Irish worriers.
Once, when a plane crashed in Europe, my grandmother panicked for days because my uncle was
on vacation in South America. Two different con-
tinents, yes, but to my grandmother, a plane was

a plane, and my uncle had been on one...which meant he could be dead.

Growing up, I was a pretty good kid. But I do remember coming home 10 minutes late from a Van Halen concert one summer. My mother was crying. She thought I was dead. Not just dead, mind you, but dead and in a ditch somewhere. Because the only thing worse than your child dead would be your child dead and in a place (a ditch?) where you'd never find her.

After 30 years of marriage, my mom even managed to spread the anxiety to my father. He called me once because a 14-year-old old Puerto Rican boy was hit by a car while walking his dog in my neighborhood. My father called to make sure it wasn't me that got hit. When I said, "Dad, you just told me that it was a 14-year-old boy from Puerto Rico, why the hell would you possibly think it might have been me??"

"He had a dog." My father answered. Ah yes, I can see how he would be nervous. I had a dog, too. !?!?

Unfortunately, I didn't escape this anxiety. I lived most of my life with a similar case of anxiety. It was never as severe, but rather it was a low-level, underlying anxiety that always had me "waiting for the other shoe to drop." If everything was going well, I waited for a catastrophe.

Misunderstandings at work led to thoughts of, *What if I lose my job?* An unreturned phone call led to thoughts of, *What if she's mad at me?* And these thoughts would quickly take on a life of their own, spinning out of control and turning from simple "what if" thoughts to thoughts of, *oh no, my life is over!* And, of course, the situation was very rarely as serious as I worried it was.

This type of anxiety is extremely common in adults with ADD. In fact, adults with ADD often find themselves with a co-existing condition, such as anxiety or depression. These conditions can be mild, severe, or somewhere in between. Either way, they wreak a lot of havoc.

One of the best things I ever did was get medication for my anxiety. If you worry so much that it affects the quality of your life (my mother and grandmother would be prime examples here), then I encourage you to get some professional help. Medication isn't for everyone, but it's worth a conversation with a good doctor. And therapists and coaches can help, too. Many therapists specialize in helping people use behavioral techniques to overcome negative thinking.

If you are a chronic worrier, the most important thing that you can do is get help. If you have anxiety or depression, then you may need professional assistance in order to help you adjust your attitude. And there's nothing wrong with this. The main goal here is that you not suffer needlessly!

Additionally, there are a few things to keep in mind when trying to change your thinking patterns. These are little changes that you can make to help you stop worrying.

1. Build Your Awareness

Notice your negative thoughts. What triggers them? What makes them worse? When you become aware of negative thoughts taking over, step back. Take a couple of really good, deep breaths. Stop what you are doing and change it up. Take a walk, get a cup of coffee, or talk to a friend. Rather than entertain a useless negative thought, force your brain to focus on something else.

2. Take Good Care of Yourself

Self-care directly affects your thinking patterns. When you're uptight and stressed, your breathing is shallow, your heart rate is faster, and your muscles are tense. In this state, it is extremely difficult to be a positive thinker, or to make any kind of positive change in your life.

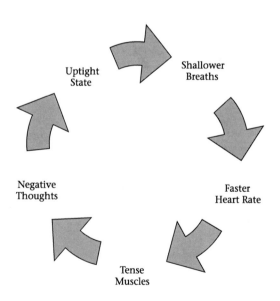

However, the opposite is also true. When you're calm and relaxed, your breathing is deeper, your heart rate is slower, and your muscles relax. In this state, your thinking patterns seem to automatically become more positive!

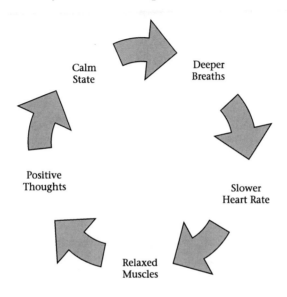

3. Surround Yourself with Happy, Positive People

Have you ever had a friend or family member who was just never happy? You know the kind: you tell them some good news and they can barely fake a moment of happiness for you before they start complaining about something. (I think we all know someone like this.)

Limit your interactions with these types of people—even if they are family. Instead, make a conscious choice to interact with positive people who are genuinely happy for your successes and supportive of your endeavors. They will lift you up and motivate you to be even more successful.

4. Get Over Perfectionism

Many ADDers don't realize that they are perfectionists, but many are! You may think that a perfectionist has it all together, but that's not the case. The hallmark of perfectionism is actually incompleteness. Perfectionists are so busy trying to make things perfect that nothing ever gets done!

Nothing is ever perfect to a perfectionist, because a perfectionist always finds something to be changed or improved. When faced with perfectionism, you must ask yourself, *would I rather that this be perfect, or done?*

If you commit to asking yourself this question, you'll soon notice just how much perfectionism slows you down and you'll learn to value "a job well done."

5. Manage Your Expectations

You and I and many others in the world have adult ADD. That means that, no matter how well you learn to manage it, you will have times in which you get overwhelmed. You will get off track. You will fall back into old patterns. But what you don't have to do is stay there!

Recognize that managing your ADD is not about curing it. It is about knowing yourself well enough to know when you aren't where you want to be...and knowing how to get back.

It's a process, and it always will be. Sure, it will get easier with time, practice, and patience. **But you will make mistakes.** Deal with it, and move on.

FORGET ABOUT OTHER PEOPLE

The second type of negative thinking comes in the form of worrying that you'll be judged by others. We're all guilty of this. Here's a good example—see if it sounds familiar.

> You attend a party with friends. Everyone is talking and laughing. You make a joke, and it flops. No one laughs and you feel stupid.
>
> You're embarrassed, so you stop participating in the conversation and just observe. You can't help thinking about how stupid you feel. Then, the host gives you a weird look...at least, you think it was a weird look, or was it?
>
> There it is again! Yes, definitely a weird look. He's pissed. You wonder, *is he mad about the joke? Did I offend him?*
>
> *Oh no, this is awful! He's mad. I bet everyone else is mad, too. Yeah, they must be. No one will even look at me!*
>
> *They must think I'm an awful person. I'll never get invited to another party as long as I live!*

This scenario happened to a client of mine. When he finally got up the courage to speak to the host of the party who gave him a "weird look," the man had no clue what he was talking about. No one was mad. Yes, the joke flopped, but it was innocent and didn't offend anyone. This client spent 2 weeks of sleepless nights worrying what his friends must think of him, and it was all in his head.

Scenarios like this are more common than you might think among adults with ADD. Fortunately, they are easy to avoid. **The key lies in separating the rational from the emotional by seeking feedback.**

Following "what if" thoughts and making assumptions about how others feel is an emotional reaction. If you allow that emotion to brood, you will fall deeper and deeper into negative thinking.

Instead, when you find yourself worried about what someone must think of you, ask them. Be rational. Explain yourself and your worries, and simply ask how the person feels. Much more often than not, you will find that your worries were unjustified, and then you can rest easy.

Every once in a while, however, you will find that someone is mad at you. Or worse yet, that they don't like you! Get over it.

Mavericks understand that some people will like you, some people will hate you, and most people will be indifferent to you. That's life. You can't win everyone over. Don't waste your time trying.

If you are true to yourself and don't hurt anyone, then who cares what other people think about you?

DUMP THE SHOULDS

If you count the number of times you say the word "should" to yourself in one day, you'll be amazed.

The word "should" often puts undue pressure on you to conform to standards that probably aren't even your own. The next time you catch yourself thinking about something that you *should* do, ask yourself if that *should* is a need to, a want to, or useless guilt.

Let's break down one particular example: *I should clean my closet.*

> **I need to clean my closet.** You threw all your tax receipts in your closet somewhere and your taxes are due! *You need to clean your closet to find those receipts and file your taxes on time.* **Make a plan to get it done.**

> **I want to clean my closet.** Your closet is a mess and it's driving you crazy! You can never seem to find what you're looking for and you're ready to change that. *You want to clean your closet to make your life easier.* **When you're ready, make a plan. Have some fun with it.**

> **I'm guilting myself about cleaning the closet.** Your closet doesn't really bother you so much. It's not the neatest closet, but you can find what you're looking for and it suits you fine. But...you just visited your friend and her closet is spotless and super organized. *You*

feel guilty because your closet isn't as nice as her closet. **Get over it and move on.**

The vast majority of "shoulds" are really just useless guilt. **The guilt results when you compare yourself to others and feel like you don't measure up.** It serves no useful purpose. It doesn't help you get things done. Instead, it knocks your self-esteem and decreases your motivation.

Remember, mavericks make their own rules! It doesn't matter if your lifestyle or systems work for other people, they only need to work for you.

Take charge of those "shoulds" and replace them with the appropriate words at every opportunity: need to, want to, or useless guilt.

Mavericks really break the rules when it comes to attitude. They don't waste time trying to be good at everything and getting down on themselves for not measuring up. Instead, they live happily and successfully by focusing on their strengths and keeping a positive demeanor.

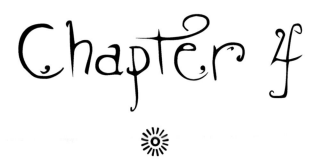

Chapter 4

Take Control of Your Space and Time

STOP TRYING TO BE SO ORGANIZED

A lack of organizational skills is probably the biggest source of pain for adults with ADD. This applies to physical spaces, as well as mental. Cluttered homes, chaotic thoughts, and mismanaged time are hallmarks of ADD in adults, and these areas often take the most time to improve upon.

Reflecting on the last chapter, mavericks understand that it's not necessary to be an expert in time management or to be super organized. Little improvements are often all you need to make a big difference in your life.

Organization and time management are the coaching meat that most ADDers are looking for. However, I take a different approach to these topics. This chapter will walk you through ADD-friendly strategies for becoming more organized and a better manager of your time. But the goal is not to fit in and be like everyone else. **The goal here is to learn what makes life easier for you, resulting in decreased stress levels and more time to enjoy yourself.**

Lisa's Story

Lisa was diagnosed with ADD at 37 after one of her kids was diagnosed. She was relieved. Lisa had always felt alone in her social network, where everyone operated so differently than she did.

Everyone else had it all together, and she didn't. Their houses were clean. Their kids were dressed neatly. Their cars were clean. They were organized. They had so many things going on—jobs, families, and volunteer work—and here was Lisa, half an hour late all the time because she could never find her car keys!

She tried so hard to do what seemed to come easily to everyone else. They accepted her, but she felt like she was inferior.

As a single mom with 4 kids, 3 dogs, 2 cats, 2 birds, and a small house, Lisa didn't throw anything away and the clutter built. She'd go into her cabinets and not recognize the labels on the soup cans because they were so old!

She was embarrassed and didn't want people coming over. She had a rule—never show up at her house unannounced. Lisa told people it was her pet peeve, but she really just wanted a chance to throw

*all the clutter in a closet before anyone came in!
When there is that much clutter, it's very difficult to clean and organize. There was tons of dust.
Between Lisa and the kids, there was always a
mountain of laundry. Plus, she had a home-based
business and no space for her office materials.*

*There came a time when her business was
going well. Lisa was respected and people really
appreciated her. People were looking to her for
direction, and asking her, "You're a single mom
with 4 kids, multiple pets, and a business—how
do you do it?"*

*Actually, Lisa didn't feel like she was "doing
it." Her home was completely disorganized! But
she felt that if all these people perceived her as
someone holding it all together, then she needed to
see herself that way, too. It was a turning point.*

*That's when Lisa found me. She knew that she
could no longer fight this battle on her own. She
knew that she needed to seek out people who could
understand her, and laugh with her about those
ADD moments.*

*Growing up, structure and organization were
provided for Lisa. Her mother was obsessed with
organization and took care of it all. She never
learned how to be organized or create structure
for herself. So when it came time to turn things
around and get organized in her own home, Lisa
wanted to involve her kids. She wanted to teach
them what she was never taught. And it really
helped her, because everyone in the household was
participating in the cleanup effort.*

They began spending a little bit of time each day decluttering the house. They got rid of the junk, and then started organizing what was left. Because they did it as a family, it was easier to stay on task. And when they got rid of all the clutter, they made room for more quality time together.

The very first day they started, they were so proud—the living room was clean! The anticipation of what needed to be done was far more overwhelming than actually digging in and cleaning up.

They're a big family in a small house, and will always have a lot of stuff. But they now know exactly how to keep it from getting out of control.

ADDers often make the mistake of thinking they can reverse years and years of difficulty by just reading a book or watching a TV show on the topic of organizing. But organization is a classic example of an area in which you may want to improve your skills, but need to be very careful not to strive for perfection. **It's time to face facts: you will probably never be an expert organizer, and you will probably never be a master of time management, either.**

Bonus Tip: It's worth mentioning that there are a number of adults with ADD who are professional organizers and well worth their fees. And some ADDers actually find that they have a real talent for organizing other people!

For adults with ADD, details are a drag. We tend

to see the big picture and want to jump straight to the finish line, wishing we could skip all the steps in between. **Organization is a problem specifically because it's all about the details.**

The solution can actually be much simpler than you think: it's all about planning. ADD mavericks don't feel the need to plan *everything*, but know that a little planning time makes a tremendous improvement in efficiency. Once the skill for planning is developed, many adults find that their lives change dramatically, and positively!

ORGANIZATION PROCRASTINATION

Before I learned about my own ADD, I frequently fell victim to *organization procrastination*. Particularly, my disorganized closets would drive me crazy. I would look for clothes to wear every morning before work and could never find what I was looking for. Clothes were hidden, and sometimes falling off the hangers. My accessories were in total disarray. And I had countless handbags piled up on the top shelf, but I never used any of them.

See if the rest of this scenario sounds familiar to you...

> One day, I'd had enough. This weekend, I decided, I was going to organize my closet... and never let it get this bad again!
> As the week went by, I would get more and more psyched. I was really going to do it this time!

Saturday came and I got up and had my coffee. I watched a little TV. I woke up fully and then decided it was time to get started. I felt good.

I cranked up the stereo. I walked into the bedroom. I opened the closet door...

...and a box fell from one of the shelves. I watched it in slow motion as it landed at my feet.

I looked up. There were tons of boxes. Lots of clothes. Things that didn't belong. And there was way too much of all of it!

I felt dizzy. I quickly slammed the closet door shut and walked out of the room. Then, I planted myself on the couch, turned on the TV, dug into some ice cream, and had a pity party.

I really wanted to clean that closet! What happened?

What happened is that I got overwhelmed, and procrastinated. And why the overwhelm? Because **I didn't know where to start**.

Organization procrastination is the result of only one thing: not having a plan.

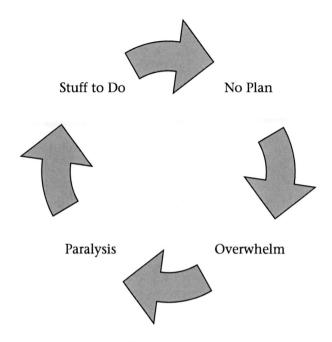

Stuff to Do — No Plan — Overwhelm — Paralysis

Jumping into a disorganized space and trying to assess all the details and make decisions on the fly causes ADD overwhelm, and overwhelm causes paralysis. The easiest way to avoid this is to plan in advance. Having a plan is akin to having a system to follow. The guesswork is removed and the stress is avoided.

PLAN THE TIME TO PLAN

Planning ahead doesn't seem like a very maverick thing to do. The truth, however, is that mavericks know and understand that without planning ahead, their goals and brilliant ideas might never see the light of day. A little planning goes a long way.

Planning is harder than it may seem for adults with ADD. It requires being calm and centered, and it requires investing some time up front. The key to planning is to step back from the situation before you begin.

Planning is a part of the organizational process and should be treated as such. Lots of adults with ADD are tempted to believe that the time required to plan is not actually work and doesn't count as time spent working towards a goal. This could not be more untrue. **Planning is a necessary step and should not be skipped.**

When making a plan, for organizing a physical space in this example, start by taking 10 minutes to sit quietly with a pen and paper. Remove yourself completely from the space you want to organize. Don't even look at the space! Then, follow these simple guidelines:

1. Determine the objective for your organizing project. What do you want to accomplish?
2. Connect with your personal motivation. Why is this goal important to you?
3. Determine 3-5 steps that you will need to complete in order to achieve your organizational goal.
4. Estimate the amount of time it will take to achieve the goal. Then, because ADDers have a poor sense of time, consider allotting double the time of your initial estimate. (The worst that

can happen is that you end up finishing early!)
5. Schedule in time to work on your project.
6. Finally, it's a good idea to schedule in maintenance time. All your hard work isn't worth much if your space becomes disorganized again in a few days.

When you craft a good plan, you take the pressure out of the organizational process. It becomes about following a system, and that's much easier to do.

> **Bonus Tip:** When determining the steps you'll need to take to complete your project, always aim for 3-5 steps. If you have less than 3 steps, then you're generalizing what has to be done and attempting to do too much in big chunks. If you have more than 5 steps, then you're either focusing too much on the details, or your project is too large. Don't start big, get overwhelmed, and find yourself paralyzed, burnt out, or bored. It's better to start small, complete a goal, and move on.

AVOID ALL OR NOTHING THINKING

One of the biggest downfalls that ADDers encounter in the organizing process is "all or nothing" thinking. All or nothing thinking means that a project is either done or not done. You've either achieved your goal, or failed. There is no in between.

One of the benefits of having a plan is that when your steps are laid out, you can easily see how close you are to completing your goal. It's easier to see shades of gray when you have a piece of paper that confirms the steps you've completed in the process.

Choose to see your progress for what it really is. Even if all you have is a plan, you've already begun and should honor the fact that you've taken steps towards achieving the goal.

FOLLOW THROUGH

It's really disheartening when you work hard to organize a space and then find that it quickly becomes disorganized again. Yet, this is exactly what happens to many adults with ADD. Clutter control is an excellent example.

The problem is one of follow through. If your plan doesn't include some solid guidelines for maintaining your space, then you'll find that the original problem doesn't take long to return.

My approach to clutter control is a little different than that of many professional organizers. I believe that in most cases, adults with ADD need to allow for clutter buildup, and also allow for clutter cleanup.

Whenever you organize a space, you need to plan on revisiting that space on a regular basis to maintain your new system. We're not the types of people that do well exclusively on the OHIO (Only Handle It Once) system. In this maintenance system, you organize as you go along, immediately putting away everything after you use it. It works well for some things, like mail, but most organizational systems will need a different plan for maintenance.

Mavericks don't worry about being neat and organized all day long. Because we don't like to be concerned with details, we often work best when we can be a little disorganized. So after decluttering a space, you may need to go about your day and not worry about it. Things might get left out or misplaced, and that's okay as long as you have a maintenance timeframe that you can adhere to. You might choose to spend 15 minutes a day, or an hour a week, on cleaning up and reorganizing. This will keep the clutter from coming back and keep the organizational systems you've created intact. As long as you have time allotted to deal with it, you won't feel pressure to organize and clean up all day.

Use This Process for All Sorts of Organizational Challenges

Physical spaces aren't the only things that need organizing. Making big decisions about your life, completing projects at work, writing a paper for a class, or determining life goals can all be made easier by stepping back and creating a plan.

When you get in the habit of taking time out to step back from the challenge and determine a plan, you'll notice that you feel a lot less stress and pressure in day-to-day life!

For more information and suggestions on clutter control and organization, visit the Odd One Out Reader's Resources webpage at **www.odd-one-out.net/resources.html**

PLAN THE TIME TO PLAN YOUR TIME

For adults with ADD, happiness in day-to-day life is largely about time management. If you start your day with a general sense of what you want to do, but without a plan for getting it all done, then chances are that you will end your day feeling stressed and frustrated.

Ben's Story

Ben is a 25-year-old Hasidic Jewish man with a wife and 3 kids. Life with ADD is very difficult in his community. He can't share his diagnosis because people won't understand. His religion doesn't permit him to have a female doctor (let alone a female coach), but he does.

Growing up in his very large family, he always felt like the odd one out. He was impulsive in school, had trouble focusing and completing assignments, and found it difficult to maintain friendships. But worse than all of that, he had no one to talk to about his challenges. No one understood. He was depressed.

When a teacher spoke to him about his pos-

sibly having ADD, Ben jumped at the chance to get a diagnosis and find out more. He had to go outside his community to do so, which was risky. He got help in the form of medication, but he was still having a lot of difficulty with work.

He was living off investment income, unsure about what to do with his time or his life. He wanted to start a business, but it wasn't working. Each day he'd wake up with no plan and jump from task to task without finishing anything. He was impulsive and regretted a lot of his decisions and actions. He wasn't getting anywhere with his business ideas, and money was running out. This put a lot of stress on his home life. His wife was worried about money, and they fought often. He felt that his life was a mess.

When Ben joined my coaching program, he found the keys he was missing. First, he had to learn how to slow down long enough to create a plan, and then he had to start planning!

Ben had never planned his time before. This was a new idea, and it soon changed everything.

Ben now has a successful real estate business. It's still a struggle sometimes, but he enjoys being in business and working toward big goals. Every night before going to sleep, he sits down and determines what he wants to do the next day. He plans in time for meditation and exercise breaks during the day so he doesn't burn out. And he leaves a little free space in his schedule in case he feels like being impulsive.

Having a daily plan takes the pressure off for

Ben. He's much more focused and he gets things done. Because of this, he comes home in a good mood at night and gets along much better with his wife. He helps out more around the house, and has more energy to enjoy time with his kids. Spending just a little time on planning makes Ben's entire day run more smoothly.

Getting your time management under control is a process. There are a number of steps that you'll have to take in order to reach the point where you don't spend your days stressed and frantic. Let's take a look at each of them, and then we'll discuss how to put it all together.

1. Choose Your Tools

In order to effectively manage your time, you're going to need some time management tools. This is a highly personalized choice and my best advice is to use what you feel comfortable with.

Don't be afraid to use a bunch of different tools in combination with each other. I use pencil and paper, monthly calendars, and a multitude of online software for scheduling and reminders. It might not make sense to anyone else, but it works for me!

Here are some ideas of time management tools that you may want to consider or experiment with:

- Daily planners (or weekly/monthly planners)
  Note: I highly recommend planners that:
  » Track a very large span of the day

> » Break time into 15-minute increments
> » Allow you to see your day and week at one glance

- Monthly calendars
- Desk calendars
- PDAs (personal, hand-held computers)
- Microsoft Outlook or other email programs with built-in time management systems
- Timers
- Various online tools designed to help with time management

For a list of free and fee-based online tools and software that I recommend, be sure to visit the Odd One Out Reader's Resources webpage at **www.odd-one-out.net/resources.html**

The one tool I absolutely insist on is a to-do list. When used properly, your to-do list is the most powerful tool in your time management arsenal.

To create your to-do list, use a pad of paper, an online program or document, or whatever feels comfortable for you.

> **Bonus Tip:** Serious mavericks may want to keep a separate list for all those "great ideas" that pop into your head that you want to accomplish someday, but don't have time for right now.

Your to-do list is a living tool. Don't let it stress you out, and don't assign any emotion to it. Your list simply helps you keep track of what you need and want to get done, as well as what you have done. You'll add things to it almost every day. And hopefully, you'll cross things off it every day, too! Your to-do list will change constantly, and it will always be necessary. Make it your friend.

2. Become Highly Familiar with Your Schedule

Have you ever been happily going about your day until you get a phone call asking why you're not where you're supposed to be—like a meeting or a doctor's appointment? When this happens, you kick yourself. You knew about the appointment, so why didn't you remember it?

As an adult with ADD, you can pretty much count on forgetting things. It's part of having attention inconsistencies. So rather than relying on your memory, you have to rely on systems.

Once you have your to-do list and other time management tools, you'll need to commit to using them every day. Yes, that's right, *every single day*! You'll need to use your time management tools diligently to record all your appointments, projects, and commitments. I realize that this sounds like hard work and may turn you off. I understand. However, if you're really serious about managing your time, this is something you'll need to commit to. I promise it's not as tedious as it sounds. All this really requires is 15 minutes a day.

First, choose a time of day in which you can consistently take 15 minutes to plan. You'll want to make sure that you choose a time in which you're alert and have a good deal of energy. Some people like to plan first thing in the morning, and some like to plan for the next day just before going to bed. Other popular planning times are mid-morning (after easing into the day) or late afternoon.

Next, you're going to tune out the rest of the world so you can focus. If you want to have some music on, that's fine, but don't let others interrupt or distract you.

Review your to-do list. Notice not just what you have to do, but also what you have actually accomplished during the day. Ceremoniously cross off or highlight your accomplishments. This step is important because it allows you to appreciate what you *did* do, thus increasing your self-esteem and motivation. Then, you may want to rewrite your to-do list, removing completed items and adding things that came up during the day. You may also want to move the most important and urgent tasks to the top of the list. And you may find it helpful to break large projects into 3-5 steps (as discussed earlier in this chapter) that all become line items on your list.

Finally, take a look at your schedule. See what appointments you have during the day. Block off the times in your schedule. Then, begin to schedule time for the tasks on your to-do list.

Bonus Tip: If you have an appointment that you need to travel to, block off the travel time in your schedule to ensure that you arrive on time!

You'll also want to block off times in which you know that you have commitments. For example, if you have to pick the kids up at 5:00 p.m., you'll want to block out 4:30–5:30 p.m. in your schedule. Similarly, if you have a daily meeting with your team at work, you'll want to block that off your schedule. If you have a commitment, make sure it's reflected in your schedule.

3. Utilize Your Time Effectively

As you review your schedule for the day, you'll notice that there are empty pockets of "free time" in your day. "Free time" is not necessarily yours to do anything you want with, but simply time you have some leeway with. This is time in which you can start knocking off the things on your to-do list.

So if you have a long list of projects at work, and you see that you have a big chunk of free time in the afternoon, you can block off that time in your schedule to work on those projects.

Instead of leaving the completion of that work up to chance, you're actually scheduling in time to get it done! You can do the same with housework and hobbies, too.

Choosing what to work on, however, may require some prioritizing. Because you have ADD, it's easy to underestimate how much time it will take for you to complete certain tasks and projects. You may set out to accomplish tons of things in a day, only to find that it's just not possible. Rather than stressing like this all the time, try looking at your to-do list and choosing just 1–3 things to work on each day. Think about what really needs to get done, and what would just be nice to get done. It may be helpful to have notes on your to-do list about deadlines.

When planning your schedule, you want to make sure that you take your natural biorhythms into account, and respect your limits.

Many ADDers take some time to ease into the day. If you're one of them, then you certainly don't want to schedule a lot of activity in the first hour or 2 after you get up. And if you are a morning person but lose steam by the end of the day, then you don't want to try and get too much accomplished in the hour or 2 before bed. It might look good on paper, but in practice it just won't work.

We all need some downtime, but what if you're at work and expected to be productive for 8 hours straight? No problem! Save the work that requires a lot of brainpower for the times that you feel the most alert and energetic, and do the work that requires less energy when you're not as alert.

For example, if you take time to ease into your day, then you may want to check your email and voicemail first thing in the morning, and save big projects for the afternoon whenever possible.

4. Schedule "Meetings with Me"

This is my favorite time management strategy and one that I utilize every chance I get.

As an adult with ADD, you're easily distracted. And if you're anything like me, you get agitated when your "flow" is interrupted.

When I worked in the corporate world, I found that late afternoon was my best time to be productive. Unfortunately, most of the office had a different biorhythm, and by that time of day many people had already put in their productive hours. They preferred meetings in the late afternoon, and I hated nothing more than a coworker showing up at my desk to chat or ask a question when I was in the middle of a productive period. It wasn't that I didn't like my coworkers; it was simply that I couldn't transition my attention from the project, to the person, and back to the project.

In order to avoid this scenario, I asked my boss if I could hang a sign on my cube wall for a few hours a day that said "Please Do Not Disturb." He agreed and it worked for a little while, but people still emailed and called during that time, which I also found distracting. And after a while, people started to ignore the sign, too. So I came up with an ingenious idea, if I do say so myself. I started scheduling "Meetings with Me."

Most offices have network calendars in which you can see whether a coworker is free for a meeting. I began blocking off time in my schedule so that it appeared to others as if I was in a meeting.

And I *was* in a meeting, with myself, doing important work.

This way, no one would try to rope me into a meeting during my productive time. If someone stopped by, I could lie (which I was fine with) and say that I had a phone meeting and I was just about to call so-and-so.

Of course, at times I had to be flexible, but for the most part it worked really well. And even though I own my own business and don't answer to anyone but myself, I still use "Meetings with Me." In fact, I'm in one right now as I write this book!

You can use "Meetings with Me" anywhere and at any time. It doesn't matter if you are an employee, a business owner, a student, or a stay-at-home parent. Whenever you need space and want to take advantage of your productive times, call a "Meeting with Me." Inform everyone that you'll be unavailable and that you are not to be interrupted. Unplug the phone. Turn the computer off. Do whatever you need to do to eliminate distractions and get some work done.

Don't be afraid to use this strategy. There is nothing mean or unreasonable about wanting to block out the distractions that can so easily knock you off course.

5. Schedule Time for Self-care

One incredible benefit of learning how to manage your time effectively is that it allows you to actually plan and schedule your self-care. This includes proper sleep, downtime, and fun time.

When taking your 15 minutes a day to plan, make sure that you schedule in your sleep time. Actually mark it down on your schedule! If you plan to go to bed at 11:00 p.m., block off about an hour before that to begin winding down. It will help ensure that your body and mind are ready for sleep, and you'll have an easier time falling asleep when you do go to bed. This goes back to Chapter 1 on breaking the cycle of overwhelm. Your wind-down time might include reading, meditating, taking a bath, or something similar.

Also, don't be afraid to schedule in some recharging time during the day. ADDers often need small periods of recharging time to remain productive and energetic throughout the day. This might include a nap, a lunch break out of the office, or even some TV time.

Lastly, take really good care of yourself by scheduling in time for your hobbies and interests. Sometimes it seems like taking a class or working on a creative project will take too much time. You may actually have to create this time in your schedule, and you should! Life is not all about being productive and accomplishing things. It's also about having fun and enjoying yourself. So when your life feels so packed that there's no time for fun, it's necessary to create that time. Be a maverick and make fun a priority.

6. Give Yourself a Weekly Check-up
Daily planning is essential, and once a week you'll
also want to give yourself a weekly check-up. This
just means that once a week, on the same day every
week, you tack a few extra minutes onto your daily
planning time so that you can review your whole
week. This is helpful for a number of reasons.

First, it gives you the opportunity to assign certain tasks to certain days. For example, perhaps
Monday is laundry day. You can then block off
a couple of hours each Monday for laundry. It
becomes a fixture in your schedule. You can do
the same for weekly meetings at work, or weekly
assignments that you're responsible for.

Second, weekly planning also allows you to
gauge your days. If you know ahead of time that
you're going to have a very busy Thursday, you
can schedule a lighter day on Friday so as not to
burn out.

During this weekly check-up, do what you
have to do to feel comfortable. You may want to
look at the coming week, or the coming month.
You can never be too familiar with your schedule
and your to-do's!

PUTTING IT ALL TOGETHER

When you learn how to manage your time effectively, your whole life will change. You'll be more
productive and you'll feel better about yourself.
You won't always be so stressed, and you'll find

that you actually have *more time* than you ever thought you did!

However, learning how to put it all together is a process. You've struggled with time management all your life, and that's not going to change overnight. It's going to take commitment and flexibility. Don't aim for perfection. You're going to screw up sometimes, so count on it! But being in control of your time sometimes is a hell of lot better than never being in control of your time. Small steps lead to big improvements.

And because putting all these steps together may seem overwhelming, I encourage you to start small and build on your successes. Begin by keeping a to-do list. When that feels comfortable, start taking 15 minutes a day to plan. Be flexible and willing to experiment. Trial and error will be a part of the process, and you are sure to find that you'll need to tweak elements of this method to fit you and your ADD. Go for it! My time management suggestions, just like the rest of this book, are simply guidelines and inspiration. What's important is that you find a way to make it work for you!

Chapter 5

✺

Live Out Loud

THE TRUE TEST OF THE MAVERICK

At this point, my friend, you're ready to get down to what really counts. You've learned how to break the cycle of overwhelm, work with your ADD, ADDjust your attitude, and take control of your space and time. You've changed your perspective about what it means to have adult ADD. And you're feeling much better about who you are and what you have to offer. It's time to start living, *really living*, for yourself. This is what being a maverick is all about: living out loud.

Living out loud is about identifying what you want in life, and believing in yourself enough to go for it. You have to stop telling yourself that your dreams are out of reach and start thinking about how to make those

dreams come to life. And in order to dream big, you have to start small.

When you live out loud, you know who you are and what you want, and you don't apologize for it. You trust yourself. You listen to your intuition. You live with intention, and you don't doubt yourself.

When you have something to say, you say it. This doesn't mean being mean or disrespectful to others; it simply means that you honor yourself, your thoughts, and your feelings.

When you want to do something, you do it. If you want to get up on stage at karaoke night, you do your thing. If you want to learn how to paint, you take a class. You don't let the doubt, judgment, or jealousy of others stop you.

There's really nothing special about adults with ADD who are successful and happy. They don't possess a magic secret that the rest of us will never get our hands on. Quite simply, they manage their ADD and live out loud. They embrace their maverick nature and make it work for them. There is absolutely no reason why you can't be a successful and happy adult with ADD who lives out loud!

Here are 3 simple guidelines to help you live out loud.

1. Never Let Fear Make Decisions for You

I can't stress this enough so I'll say it again: **NEVER LET FEAR MAKE DECISIONS FOR YOU!**

Fear is a normal human emotion, and fear serves a very useful purpose. It helps keep us in check. It helps ensure that we make good decisions. But when it comes to living out loud, fear should never be the only thing that you consider when making a decision.

Living out loud requires you to take risks, both big and small. And risks involve fear.

Risk taking is not thrill seeking. We're not talking about engaging in dangerous behavior. We're simply talking about stretching your comfort zone. This means that you are willing to endure some uncomfortable feelings or situations in order to achieve the things you want.

Risks *are* uncomfortable, but they have the potential to be rewarding. Let's look at some examples.

If you work really hard at your job and you know that you're not being paid as much as you're worth, then asking for a raise is a risk. It's scary. There's a chance you'll be rejected. But there is also a chance that you'll be rewarded. Only one thing is certain: if you don't actually take the risk and ask for the raise, you'll continue being underpaid.

If you live out loud, you might schedule a meeting with your boss to talk about this problem, then very confidently detail the reasons why you deserve that raise. If you get it, the risk paid off! If you don't get it, then you may decide that in order to live out loud, it's time to look for a new job.

When I was 25, I found out that I was being underpaid compared to some of the other people in my department. I knew I was valuable to the company and I was pissed. I followed the process above and asked for a $15,000 raise. I got it *that day.*

Similarly, if you've always wanted to paint, but never learned how for fear of embarrassing yourself, then taking a class is a risk. The idea of not being as good as those around you is scary. If you push through that fear, you may find that you actually have a hidden talent! Or you may find that you aren't talented at all when it comes to painting, but really enjoy it anyway! If you never take the class, then you'll always regret never finding out.

Feeling fear is okay. In fact, it's healthy! But fear becomes a problem if it stops you from achieving—or even attempting to achieve—your goals.

If the fear of failure, rejection or judgment stops you in your tracks, then you're not living out loud. Take your fear into account when making your decisions, but never let it make your decisions for you. **If you let it take over, fear will forever keep you from reaching your potential.**

2. Expect Failure

My Story

When I was new to the coaching field, I often heard people say, "There is no such thing as failure. Everything is a learning experience."

I didn't buy it. In my view, losers failed. Winners did not even entertain the idea of failure.

Early on in my coaching career I decided to

put together a 90-day group coaching program designed to teach the Essential Skills. I was really excited about it because I wanted to do some group coaching. I had some great material, and I was eager to present it in a structured format. And I knew that a group of peers working towards common goals often carries an individual further than a private coaching experience.

At the time I was preparing for the group, I was renting a small office one day a week in New York City. I saw a few clients privately and ran a few support groups. I invited those clients to join the group. I put fliers in my office waiting room and gave some to all the mental health professionals I knew. I had the group added to local events guides. And, of course, I announced the event multiple times to my email newsletter subscribers. But no one was signing up.

A couple of weeks before the group was scheduled to start, I was freaking out. I spoke to my business coach at the time, Chris Barrow of the UK-based Dental Business School, and told him what was going on. I was afraid that I wouldn't be able to make this group thing work, even though I really wanted to.

In a 15-minute conversation, I got the best lesson of my life. Chris said to me, "...so you keep promoting the group, and if you fail—"

"Whoa, Chris, hang on!" I interrupted him. "The word "fail" is not in my vocabulary. I do not fail."

Chris didn't skip a beat. "Well you will fail.

And you better get used to it, because it will happen a lot." My forehead was crinkling on the other end of the phone. I didn't like what I heard.

"And when you do fail," he continued in a very matter-of-fact tone, "you will get right back up. You'll do what you can to figure out what you did wrong, and then you'll be one step closer to success."

*I was resistant to this idea at first, but once that seed was planted, everything changed. I actually added the word "fail" to my vocabulary, and I stopped thinking about it as a bad thing. **I stopped being afraid of it.***

And once I stopped being afraid of failure, suddenly nothing was impossible. I felt like I had permission to put myself out there, in a big way, because if it didn't work, then it didn't work. So what?

I started to see failure as something that happened to everyone, not an indicator that I sucked at what I was doing. And I don't just rely on this knowledge anymore, I live by it.

Incidentally, I ended up with 5 people in that coaching group. I guess I took it for granted at the time that ADDers don't do many things early, and that includes registering for coaching programs!

One of the reasons that adults with ADD don't live out loud and embrace the maverick within is they're afraid of failure. It's time to change your perspective on failure.

If you're going to live out loud, you can't be afraid of failure. You have to accept it, and even expect it, as a part of life.

Just like everyone else in the world, we sometimes succeed at what we set out to do, and sometimes we don't. And when you don't succeed, the worst thing you can do is beat yourself up about it.

So many successful adults with ADD feel like frauds. We tend to be extremely hard on ourselves. No matter what you do, you could be doing it better. No matter how much you do, you could be doing more. It might be good enough for everyone else, but it's never good enough for you.

Holding yourself to high standards can work to your advantage because it can help you push forward when things get tough. **But when the standards become impossible and you have to get it right on the first try, you're not allowed to screw up, and you have to be _the_ best, then those standards are no longer serving you, they're defeating you.**

You won't always get it right the first try. You will screw up. And you won't always be the best. So if you tell yourself the opposite, and can't attain these impossible feats, then of course you'll feel like a fraud.

We all do the best we can with the skills and tools we have available to us. No one sets out to fail. So what's the point of beating yourself up? What good does it do? Getting down on yourself never helps relieve your stress or solve your problems. It only makes things worse—much, much worse.

The better solution is to make a choice to move forward. Failure is really a form of feedback. When trying to achieve a goal, you may fail many times. And each time you fail, you're given a piece of the puzzle you're trying to solve. Knowing what doesn't work only brings you closer to finding out what will.

Lots of things will get in the way of you achieving your goals. Don't be one of them.

Bonus Tip: Winners do quit, and quitters do win.

I'd like to meet the jerk who coined the phrase "winners never quit and quitters never win." It's the biggest load of bullshit that's ever been fed to us.

Real winners know when it's time to stop working towards unrealistic goals. Real winners know that quitting is not a sign of weakness.

Real winners make informed decisions about when it's time to keep pushing, and when it's time to quit.

3. Turn Your Dreams into Goals

Dreaming is easy. Creating plans to achieve those dreams is much harder. But that's one of the things that people who live out loud do really well. They identify the dreams that are most important to them, and they take concrete steps towards achieving those dreams.

First and foremost, you have to believe that you are capable of achieving your dreams. You may never be a rock star, but you can learn some skills, play in a band, and taste your dream.

You may never be able to afford a yacht, but with some work and determination, you could buy a pleasure boat. Or you could take a lavish vacation on a yacht.

You may never be President of the United States, but you could be a local or state politician and still make a very big difference.

So what's stopping you?

Most people think that a lack of money is what's stopping them from achieving their dreams. That's an excuse.

Our dreams are never really about money; they're about the lifestyles that we would live if we had a lot of money. We all think that money would bring with it toys, freedom, and happiness. And I'm sure it would! But you can have toys, freedom, and happiness without winning the lottery. You just need to identify exactly what it is that you feel like you're missing in your life—you need to really examine your dreams to find out—and then begin working towards achieving those things here and now.

Money is not what stops people from achieving their dreams. Confidence and the lack of a plan are really what stop people. You deserve to have everything that you want in life. **You deserve to define success and happiness for yourself, and you deserve to achieve success and happiness on your own terms.** This is a basic human right, and one that adults with ADD so often rob themselves of simply because they think they don't deserve it!

If you're going to be a maverick and live out loud, then you need to convince yourself, right here and now, that you deserve it. You deserve to take those dreams and turn them into reality.

START LIVING OUT LOUD TODAY

Working towards your dreams is not as hard as you might think. You've already learned how to break a project down into steps and manage your time effectively to achieve those goals. Now you just have to take that knowledge and apply it to the big picture of your life.

Start by determining what you want in your life. Not necessarily what things you want in your life, but what elements you want in your life. Do you want more freedom? Do you want to work less? Spend more time with your family? Travel the world? Be more creative? Explore your talents? Think about it. And if you really want that expensive sports car or that vacation home, well then, my friend, live out loud and go for it!

Create a clear vision of what you want to achieve. Journal about it, daydream about it, and maybe even share it with a supportive person in your life. When you know what it is that you want, you can start working towards achieving it. Jump ahead and work backwards. Ask yourself where you want to be a year from now, and then take some time to plan some steps.

Figure out what you can do in the next year to work towards your goal, then figure out what you can do in the next 6 months, the next 3 months, the next week, and even tomorrow!

Dreams don't come true unless you make them come true. And when your dreams come true, you're living out loud. You're embracing the maverick you were meant to be.

Conclusion

Success and Happiness on Your Terms

WHAT IT REALLY MEANS TO MANAGE YOUR ADD

I've worked with quite a few coaches. When looking for a coach, whether in my personal life or my business life, I always look for someone who has "been there and done that." Someone who understands the situation that I'm in and what it's going to take for me to move to the next level.

I don't want to work with someone who's perfect and has it all figured out. I want to work with someone who lives out loud and continually strives for the next level, just like I do. I want to work with someone who has challenges, and overcomes them. I want to work with someone who is real, because that's who I know I can learn the most from.

So I can relate when my own clients ask about my ADD. *Do you ever run late? Do you miss deadlines? Do you get distracted and lose focus?*

Hell yes!

Successfully managing your ADD is *not* about eliminating your ADD challenges. Here's what it *is* about:

- It's about learning how to manage your ADD most of the time.
- It's about knowing when you need help getting back on track.
- It's about noticing when you've been sidetracked, and knowing how to get back to where you need to be.
- It's about understanding that you will have challenges, but they don't need to bring you down or get in the way of you achieving your goals.

My hope for you is that you will take the information, strategies, and inspiration from this book and use them to your advantage.

My hope for you is that you create your own definitions of success and happiness, and that you achieve them for yourself.

My hope for you is that you embrace the person you are—ADD and all—and move forward in your life with pride and confidence.

Live successfully. Live happily. Be a maverick. And never be afraid to be the odd one out.

ODD ONE OUT READER'S RESOURCES

Don't forget to visit the Odd One Out Reader's Resources webpage at:

www.odd-one-out.net/resources.html

Note: Depending on your web browser, you may need to type:
http://www.odd-one-out.net/resources.html
to access the page.

On the Reader's Resources webpage, you'll find helpful recommendations for:

- Additional reading
- Online and offline time management tools
- Links to informational articles and studies
- Coaching programs and services offered by my company, the ADD Management Group
- Coaching products and next steps for going deeper into the subjects covered in this book

www.odd-one-out.net/resources.html